THE PATIENT'S GUIDE TO PREVENTING MEDICAL ERRORS

THE PATIENT'S GUIDE TO PREVENTING MEDICAL ERRORS

Karin Janine Berntsen

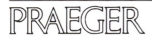

Westport, Connecticut
London

Berntsen, Karin Janine.
    The patient's guide to preventing medical errors / Karin Janine
Berntsen.
        p. cm.
    Includes bibliographical references and index.
    ISBN 0–275–98230–0 (alk. paper)
    1. Medical errors—United States—Prevention.   I. Title.
R729.8.B476 2004
    610—dc22   2004040052

British Library Cataloguing in Publication Data is available.

Library of Congress Catalog Card Number: 2004040052
ISBN: 0–275–98230–0

First published in 2004

Praeger Publishers, 88 Post Road West, Westport, CT 06881
An imprint of Greenwood Publishing Group, Inc.
www.praeger.com

Printed in the United States of America

The paper used in this book complies with the
Permanent Paper Standard issued by the National
Information Standards Organization (Z39.48–1984).

10   9   8   7   6   5   4   3   2   1

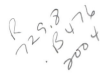

Copyright Acknowledgments

Every reasonable effort has been made to trace the owners of copyright materials in this book, but in some instances this has proven impossible. The author and publisher will be glad to receive information leading to more complete acknowledgments in subsequent printings of the book, and in the meantime extend their apologies for any omissions.

The author and publisher gratefully acknowledge permission to reprint the following:

Material from the Joint Commission on Accredidation of Healthcare Organizations website. Copyright © Joint Commission on Accredidation of Healthcare Organizations, 2003. Reprinted with permission.

Excerpts from "The Wrong Patient" by Chassin and Beecher, *Annals of Internal Medicine*, 2002, 136: 826–833. Reprinted with the permission of the American College of Physicians.

Tips and Information in: *The Patient's Guide to Preventing Medical Errors*

A warning: The information in this book is NOT intended as medical advice. These tips are intended *only* to be helpful and used as a commonsense approach and guide to avoiding medical errors.

For any concerns, questions, uncertainties, medical advice, or unusual situations, contact your physician. For any emergency, call 911.

These tips are NOT intended to be all-inclusive with regard to the prevention of all medical or medication errors.

"Be strong . . . and work, for I am with you," says the Lord of Hosts.
Haggai 2:4

This book is dedicated to the memory of my dear mother, Janine, and to my special husband, Alan, and my extraordinary son, Jonathan.

CONTENTS

Photo essay follows chapter 8.

ACKNOWLEDGMENTS

I want to acknowledge the people, particularly the children, who have been harmed by medical errors. Hospitals were designed to heal, to help the infirm and sick recover and return to a healthy lifestyle. Great advancements in medicine have accomplished many wonders and have brought healing to countless people. Nevertheless, with no malicious intent, some hospitals have harmed rather than healed people.

By writing this book for the general public, I hope to lessen the chance that medical errors will occur. The stories I have shared about patients and their families or one of the tips provided here may encourage readers to be extra careful, stop, speak up, and ask questions, all good strategies that may help to identify circumstances that lead to errors. My hope is that this information alerts people everywhere to be more involved in their health care.

I thank those who have spoken up about their medical errors, those who were willing to share stories of their suffering so that other people might avoid a similar circumstance. Additionally, I acknowledge the health care professionals who are working hard for the cause of patient safety and who have been my colleagues and friends in this endeavor. I thank Willa Fields for first teaching me the principles of quality whereby all improvements, including patient safety, are made; Louise Balesteri for her dedicated support and literally being my right-hand person over the years; Michael Long, M.D., for his dedicated support to the cause of quality; Annette Graham, whose intelligence in health care matters is unsurpassed; Wendy Kaler, who battles every day to prevent and control infectious diseases; Marcia Hall for her guidance and support over the years; Holly Heaton for her dedication to a fair and balanced approach to legal health care issues; Michele Tarbet for her support and leadership; Robert Pachorek for his promotion of medication safety; and Gerrie James, my friend and spiritual supporter, who said, "You can do this!"

In addition, I thank Michael, whose intelligence and past experience in receiving medical care helped to encourage me to persevere with this important endeavor.

And last, I acknowledge my many staff members over the years who have been diligent and faithful in helping to improve patient care every day.

INTRODUCTION

It is natural to feel apprehensive when facing a surgical procedure or entering a hospital to receive treatment for a newly diagnosed illness. Although a bit nervous, people assume that they will be safe. That assumption is wrong. A startling report revealed that it is far safer to fly on a commercial airliner than to be a patient in a hospital. In fact, receiving health care services is considered as dangerous as mountain climbing or bungee jumping.

The extensive report, "To Err Is Human: Building a Safer Health System," from the Institute of Medicine (IOM) in Washington, D.C., states that up to 98,000 people die each year as a result of medical errors in U.S. hospitals. This is equivalent to 268 fatalities a day, or the loss of a fully loaded 767 airliner. Numerous others suffer from injuries while hospitalized, ranging from minor falls to permanent disability. The IOM report reveals that over half of these deaths and injuries are preventable.[1]

Medical errors need to be significantly decreased. The "error factor" occurring in health care systems is complex, multifactorial, and challenging to solve. Faulty systems that lead to patient injury and death should be identified and new, safer systems designed. However, changes in these intricate systems will happen more effectively and rapidly only with the involvement of health care consumers. There is a need for a professional-public partnership to be forged in order to work together for solutions. If patients can learn about health care system vulnerabilities, and, most importantly, if they can learn to be more involved in their care, then perhaps some medical errors may be avoided. As with other circumstances, knowledge is power; moreover, knowledge of vulnerable health care systems and the medical errors that take place within them may be the means to help save lives.

Debbie, for example, developed diabetes when she was 14 and required several injections of insulin each day. Recently she developed the flu and went to the emergency room with a slightly elevated blood sugar level. She normally administered her own insulin but was feeling too ill to do so. The nurse caring for Debbie came in with a syringe of insulin. The nurse placed the insulin syringe into Debbie's intravenous (IV) line port. Even though Debbie was feeling poorly, she glanced over at the syringe and screamed "Stop!" The doctor had written an order for 10 units of a fast-acting insulin, but the nurse was about to inject 100 units in error. The syringe markings were small and the nurse had misread them. This overdose of insulin would have killed Debbie within minutes of the injection. What prevented this error from having fatal consequences? Debbie was thoroughly knowledgeable about her diabetes and specifically the medication required to treat her illness. A less aware patient might not have been so fortunate.

Throughout a 25-year career in health care, I have witnessed many near misses and encountered serious medical errors as well. Most recently, as vice president of patient safety and quality improvement for a seven-hospital health care system in southern California, I reviewed significant medical errors from both preventive and medical-legal perspectives.

As a registered nurse and former paramedic specializing in trauma, emergency medicine, and cardiac care, which included other roles as emergency cardiac coordinator, telemetry unit manager, state nurse educator, and nursing director, I recognize that health care services are fragmented and prone to error. I was moved by "To Err Is Human" and am relieved that an official report substantiates my observation—that too many people are being harmed by preventable medical errors.

The IOM report quickly moved hospital leaders into action—participating in national conferences, creating patient safety plans, collecting data, and implementing patient safety projects. All of these initiatives are steps in the right direction. Clearly, health care leaders have developed the passion needed to change the equation of harm.

Yet, as I lead hospital safety committees, coordinate patient safety seminars, teach on the reduction of medical errors and research best practices—which were all designed to reduce medical errors—I consistently note that patients are not at the core of this new culture change. I have been troubled by the fact that hospital professionals are failing to work with the public to design safer systems. I also recognized that strategies to involve consumers are complex. How do we ask patients about medical error prevention without frightening them? How do we collect and incorporate consumer ideas into safety planning when consumers do not understand the intricacies of complicated health systems? Will soliciting public involvement slow the progress that we as professionals need to accomplish?

These questions led me to review the literature on safety resources available to the public. I found a myriad of information on reducing medical errors designed for professionals, but very little targeted for the consumer. Moreover, there was little material that focused on formulating error-prevention partnerships with the public.

In writing this book, I hope to inform consumers about the problem of medical errors and begin to forge the *partnership of change.* I selected real stories based on illustrations of health care system vulnerabilities as opposed to those that target individual blame. Even though numerous other stories could be shared, these illustrations reveal the complexity of interactions that are built into health care systems and allow for medical errors.

The situations described in these accounts have occurred and continue to occur in U.S. hospitals. Some of the stories in this book use the patients' actual names, because they have been willing to publish their experiences. Other names, times, and places have been changed to protect patient identities. Some events occur repeatedly within hospitals, and key factors of several cases have been combined to illustrate common hospital system breakdowns.

This book focuses primarily on the hospital experience, with some examples of outpatient settings and doctors' offices included to help illustrate health care system vulnerabilities. Additional research is warranted on the outpatient setting, physicians' offices, and long-term-care facilities, given that the problem of medical errors is not isolated to hospitals.

Although I have chosen to write about the vulnerability of health care systems, I do not address the complex problem of the nursing shortage. This problem alone warrants an exploration of the many issues surrounding this critical situation as well as potential solutions. The nursing shortage has no doubt had an impact on system breakdowns; however, this book is written to address the broader problem of failed health care systems and to move the consumer to action.

With all this in mind, the consumer needs to demand changes in health care. Since the IOM report, there has been little consumer pressure on legislative bodies to reduce medical errors and improve health care systems. This may be due in part to the fact that consumers do not have ongoing, relevant information on medical errors. The public knows there is a problem, yet the means to help people take steps toward error reduction is lacking. Almost without exception, each person I have told that I was researching and writing this book described to me a friend or family member who had a medical mishap. Even with these experiences, people felt a lack of empowerment to change fragmented health care systems.

Until safer systems are designed, patients and families must take a leading role in driving what happens to them while they are receiving health care services. Patients should move away from blind trust and begin speaking up and avoiding assumptions of safety. Often people feel intimidated or rushed when they have questions for clinicians. Other times people feel they are at the disposal of a surgeon or specialist and are careful not to "make the doctor mad" because they have to receive ongoing treatment from that practitioner. Ultimately, this culture needs to shift into a patient-centered model. This book is written as a guide to help consumers make this shift by giving them information so they feel more confident and less intimidated in speaking up about their concerns.

Last, and just as significant, the book provides practical resources in the form of consumer tips and information on referral organizations. By using these resources, the public can gain the knowledge needed to maneuver through the complex medical system and possibly to prevent errors from occurring.

CHAPTER 1

THE ERROR FACTOR

JESICA

On February 7, 2003, Jesica Santillán was scheduled for a heart-lung transplant. Jesica was looking forward to receiving her new heart and lung. The thought of feeling better, not having fainting spells, and having more energy excited her.

The doctors assured the Santilláns that Jesica was an excellent candidate for the transplant. Jesica was 17 and had her whole life to look forward to. She had been born with a heart defect and was small for her age, only 90 pounds. This transplant was a chance for a new beginning. After all, Duke University Hospital was one of the leading hospitals in the country. A few years earlier, the Santilláns had come from Mexico to the United States in order to receive the best care for Jesica.

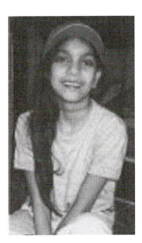

Jesica Santillán

After surgery, when Jesica was removed from the heart bypass machine, something began to go terribly wrong. Jesica's vital signs were not responding the way they should have been, and the operating room team had to put her back on cardiac bypass. The new organs were not functioning. Shortly after the OR team realized that Jesica was in trouble, a call came from the laboratory. Jesica's blood was incompatible with that of her new heart and lung. Jesica had O positive blood and the

Table 1.1
How Safe Is Health Care?

Less than 1 death per 100,000 encounters
Nuclear power

European railroads

Scheduled airline flights

One death in less than 100,000 but more than 1,000 encounters
Driving

Chemical manufacturing

More than 1 death per 1,000 encounters
Bungee jumping

Mountain climbing

Health care

Source: Richard Smith (ed.). (2001). *British Medical Journal.*

> *organ donor was type A. This combination causes the most severe form of a*
> *blood reaction.*
>
>   *Although an attempt was made to reverse the blood reaction and Jesica*
> *was given a new heart and lung, it was too late. By February 21, 2003, the*
> *doctors realized that Jesica had irreversible brain damage. Jesica died on*
> *February 22, 2003.*

What Went Wrong?

Jesica died as a result of a hemolytic blood reaction. The official autopsy report stated, "Given the historical circumstances and the autopsy findings, it is my opinion that this young woman's death was the result of global cerebral hypoxic injury that was a complication of the rejection of an . . . incompatible heart-lung transplant." The report was signed by Dr. John Butts, the chief state medical examiner in North Carolina.[1]

Hemolytic reactions are rare. When they do occur they are very serious and can be fatal. This reaction is also known as ABO incompatibility. Jesica's blood, type O, had no ability to handle blood cells with type A antigens. Antibodies within her blood plasma would attack either a type A or a type B donor's blood cells.

Often a hemolytic reaction can lead to a condition known as disseminated intravascular coagulation (DIC). DIC is a problematic and complex condition that starts with microscopic bleeding and eventually leads to an overreaction of the body's blood clotting system. Tiny blood clots develop throughout the body and ultimately lead to lack of oxygen for vital organs, including the brain (as occurred with Jesica). Kidney failure, heart failure, and death ensue.

Because a surgeon is technically in charge of the surgical case, Dr. James Jaggers, Jesica's transplant surgeon, assumed accountability for the organ mix-up. Conversely, he is not fully responsible for it. No one person, no human error alone is to blame. The medical error that took Jesica's life was the result of system design failures.

Just after the error occurred, Duke University Hospital released the following letter. This letter helps to identify the components of the "error factor" and illustrates the complex methods and multiple steps involved in most health care processes that allow for medical errors to occur.

From: Duke University Hospital
February 21, 2003
To: United Network for Organ Sharing (UNOS)

Dear ___ :

Duke University Hospital has completed the initial phase review of the events related to the heart/lung transplant from donor ___. We provide the following to promote our joint efforts in the peer review of this incident and for the purpose of performance improvement.

We have concluded that human error occurred at several points in the organ placement process that had no structured redundancy. The critical failure was absence of positive confirmation of ABO compatibility of the donor organs and the identified recipient patient. The transplant surgeon does not recall receiving or requesting information regarding the donor's ABO type from the procurement coordinator, who released the organs for the specific recipient.

Jesica Santillán . . . was then listed for heart/lung transplantation in May 2002.

An offer from Carolina Donor Services (CDS) of organs was made in the evening on 2/6/03. The organs were offered to Dr. A., the adult heart transplant surgeon on call, for a pediatric heart transplant recipient. Because the potential recipient was a pediatric patient, Dr. A. referred CDS to Dr. B., the pediatric heart transplant surgeon on call.

Dr. B. declined for the specified patient because that patient was not ready for transplant. Dr. B. inquired about heart/lung availability for Jesica Santillán, specifying the patient by name. Dr. B. inquired about the status of the lungs. The organ procurement coordinator stated that he would check this and call back.

On the return call, Dr. C., the lung and heart/lung adult transplant surgeon on call, then was offered a heart/lung block from this donor for an adult recipient. He declined due to size incompatibility. The organs were then offered by CDS to Dr. B. for Jesica Santillán.

Dr. B. accepted the offer. He does not recall ABO typing being discussed with CDS but does recall a discussion of height, weight, and cause of death. Arrangements were made for Jesica Santillán to be admitted to the Pediatric ICU and for the harvest team to travel to the donor site to retrieve the organs.

On arrival at the donor site, the harvesting physician, Dr. D., examined the organs of the donor and reviewed the donor packet. Dr. D. judged the organs to be of good quality. He called Dr. B. and reported the condition of the organs and was directed to harvest the heart and lungs. The organs were transported back to Duke University Hospital following a delay due to bad weather.

Once the organs arrived at the Duke University Hospital operating room No. 7, the recipient's heart and lungs were removed and the donor organs were implanted . . .

. . . The organs functioned well for approximately 30–40 minutes after she was removed from bypass. Then the organ function deteriorated, and the patient was placed back on cardiopulmonary bypass.

Moments later, the OR received a call from the Duke University Hospital Clinical Transplant Immunology Laboratory reporting the transplant was ABO incompatible with the recipient . . .

. . . In response, Duke University Hospital has conducted a thorough root cause analysis of the event and the organ procurement process followed in the pediatric thoracic transplant program. During that review, the lack of redundancy was recognized as a weakness. Validation of the ABO compatibility and other key data elements regarding the donor and recipient will now be performed by:

• the transplant surgeon
• the transplant coordinator, and
• the procuring surgeon.

The transplant surgeon will actively confirm the donor and recipient key data elements verbally.

During the notification call to the transplant surgeon, the donor key data elements will be communicated. These data elements will be compared to the information in the transplant program's database to confirm blood type compatibility, size compatibility and if there are issues regarding anti-HLA antibodies.

An additional verification will be accomplished via telephone contact with the organ procurement organization placement coordinator by the transplant coordinator. The procuring surgeon will receive information including, but not limited to the ABO type and size about the intended recipient.

In the review of the donor packet, the procuring surgeon will verify the ABO compatibility as well as other key elements used to evaluate the suitability of the donor and the organs for the targeted recipient.

In addition, the procuring surgeon will complete a verbal verification of the ABO compatibility with the transplant surgeon. This call will be placed, as per current standard, prior to the organ procurement.

The verification processes outlined above were effectively implemented during the re-transplant of the recipient of [second] donor's ___ organs on February 20, 2003.

In addition to the redundant validation put in place, Duke University Hospital is evaluating the information technology supporting access to recipient information. Should that evaluation reveal a need for additional support, resources will be dedicated to meet those needs. We will continue to examine the organ procurement process for opportunities for additional safeguards. We will monitor the effectiveness of the process changes through our performance improvement program.

We believe that the changes we have put in place enhance the safety of the procurement process and should be considered as a national guideline.

Should you require additional information please do not hesitate to contact us.

Sincerely,

———— 2

Events such as these happen in U.S. hospitals too frequently. It is clear in this multistep process, with the health care system's reliance on memory, lack of protocols, many hand-offs, and lack of technology support, that there are numerous opportunities for mistakes to occur.

Tragically, as this story plays out, the system failures that resulted in Jesica's death are not unusual. Several other case examples will be discussed throughout this book to specifically illustrate the type of system failures that commonly occur in health care.

What Are the Facts?

The Institute of Medicine (IOM), founded in 1970 through the National Academy of Sciences (an organization established by Congress), published an extensive report in 1999, "To Err Is Human: Building a Safer Health System."[3] The IOM report states that between 44,000 and 98,000 Americans die each year as a result of medical errors, accelerating the death rate above that of motor vehicle accidents (43,358), breast cancer (42,297), and AIDS (16,516). This report reveals that 3.7 percent of hospital patients end up with a disabling injury inflicted by medical care from an adverse event. The report further outlines that between 6.6 and 13.6 percent of adverse events occurring to patients result in death. Astoundingly, half of the deaths are preventable.

The IOM report lists various types of errors that occur within hospitals. These include transfusion errors, adverse drug events, wrong site or side surgery, surgical injuries, hospital-acquired infections, falls, burns, restraint-related injuries, and fractures.[4]

Tips

When you are receiving health care services, *you* can be the most important factor in preventing an error from affecting you.

Beware that errors can occur in any hospital or health care setting.

The Harvard Study

To establish the conclusions regarding errors, the IOM reviewed results from the Harvard Medical Practice Study, which looked at more than 30,000 randomly selected patient discharges from 51 hospitals in New York State. The study's findings were projected over the 33.6 million admissions to United States hospitals during 1997.[5] In combination with the Harvard study, the IOM reviewed over 15,000 patient records from Colorado and Utah. This research examined errors that occurred inside and outside of hospitals and found that four out of five errors happened while the patient was in the hospital. In fact, the hospital setting is prone to the highest number of errors.

Nevertheless, the consumer should not ignore the fact that significant errors can occur in physicians' offices and other nonhospital settings, such as clinics, outpatient centers, and nursing homes. The number of studies done in outpatient settings, however, is limited and needs further research. In addition to these two large studies, the IOM also reviewed 30 other studies on medical errors, which were also a basis of its conclusions regarding deaths from medical errors.[6]

Tips on Blood Products

Most blood that is administered comes in the form of blood products, such as packed (concentrated) red blood cells (RBCs), or other components of whole blood, such as plasma. These products use the part of the whole blood that will benefit the patient the most. Whole blood can be overwhelming for the body to assimilate and it is rarely transfused, except for special illnesses. Ask, "Am I receiving red blood cells, plasma, or other parts of blood?" Be sure you understand the kind of blood or blood products you will be receiving.

The risk for an acute hemolytic transfusion reaction (AHTR) is 1:25,000 with the risk of a fatal reaction at 1:160,000.[7]

When receiving blood or blood products, have a thorough discussion with your doctor about the reason you are receiving blood, including the results of any blood tests that are guiding the doctor to make the decision for you to receive them.

If you receive blood or blood products, you should know your own blood type—A, B, AB, or O—as well as whether your blood is Rh positive or Rh negative (Rh factor). Ensure that you or a family member confirms that the blood you receive is the same blood type as your own.

When signing your consent for surgery, read it thoroughly to see if it includes a clause regarding consent for blood administration. Some hospitals combine these consents, and you should be aware that you might receive blood if needed.

BEN KOLB

A Case of Death by Medication Error

In December 1995 at a Florida hospital, Ben Kolb, age seven, was scheduled for elective ear surgery at Martin Memorial Hospital. Ben had a history of ear problems and had already undergone two successful ear surgeries, one

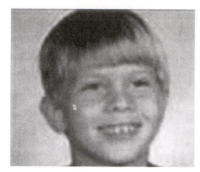

Ben Kolb

when he was two years old and one when he was five. This surgery was expected to be another routine procedure.

It was two weeks before Christmas. Tammy and Tim, Ben's parents, were looking forward to the holidays. Tim was very proud of his son and enjoyed coaching Ben's soccer team. Ben, a natural-born leader, was the team's captain.

Ben was taken to surgery.

After Ben was taken to the operating room, the surgeon's first step was to administer lidocaine to numb the surgical area around Ben's ear. The syringe that the surgeon believed contained lidocaine, however, was filled instead with epinephrine. Within seconds of the injection, Ben's heart rate soared, and he went into cardiac arrest. Even though the operating room team worked for two hours to revive Ben, he slipped into a coma and died within 24 hours of the injection.[8]

Across the United States, all hospitals are fundamentally designed the same; hence errors that occur at one hospital can be common to all hospitals. Health systems are complex, with many forms of communication. The workflow occurs in such a way that many duties are handed off and interchanged among doctors, nurses, and other members of the health care team. These handoffs increase the chance of errors occurring.

How did two completely different drugs that create such opposite effects become mixed up during surgery? A later investigation of what went wrong in Ben Kolb's case revealed vulnerabilities in the system design of the operating room processes. Design flaws consisted of multiple latent (hidden) conditions that were present in the process for a number of years, setting up the system for failure and leading to Ben's death.

A nurse in the operating room on the day of Ben's surgery removed two medications from their original containers and placed the drugs in two separate cups. Routinely, lidocaine, which is injected to numb an area, was always placed in a metal cup and epinephrine (adrenaline), which is intended only for use on top of the skin, was placed in a plastic cup. The cups were then placed next to each other on an operating room table. This procedure had been carried out hundreds of times before in the Martin Memorial Hospital operating rooms and thousands of times more in operating rooms across the United States.

In Ben's case, a different nurse took a syringe and drew up the medicine from the metal cup that she thought contained lidocaine. Unknown to this nurse, the epinephrine had accidentally been placed in the metal cup. Both medicines are clear liquids that are indistinguishable from each other. The surgeon, who thought he had the lidocaine, injected the epinephrine surrounding Ben's ear. Epinephrine injected in this concentration causes a massive reaction and overstimulation of the body's vital organs—conditions that led to Ben's death.

Processing the medications in this manner was a faulty system design fraught with hidden conditions. It was only a matter of time until something went wrong. Tragically, this time the Kolb family paid the price. Broken processes and systems such as this exist too frequently in U.S. hospitals.

After the devastating error, Martin Memorial Hospital overhauled its operating room process. The leaders put in double and triple checks so that this error could not recur. Nonetheless, there was no mandate, regulation, or guarantee that the medical error with Ben Kolb's case had to be widely shared with other hospitals. Therefore, this same error could still occur today.

Injury from Adverse Events

The number of people who die as a result of adverse events is certainly alarming; additionally, injuries and disability from medical errors is a significant concern. In the Harvard study, 2.6 percent of adverse events resulted in permanent disability. The IOM reviewed another study that looked at 815 adverse events in patients from a university hospital. The study showed that of the 815 incidents, 9 percent were an iatrogenic illness that threatened life or resulted in a significant disability. Iatrogenic is a term that describes an event that results from a diagnostic procedure, a therapy, or a harmful event that was not part of the patient's condition. Another revealing fact from the IOM report showed that the chance of an adverse event occurring increased with each added day of hospitalization, an increased risk of 6 percent each day.[9] Hence, the longer a person is hospitalized, the greater his or her risk for a medical error.

The Impact of Errors

According to an article published in the *Journal of the American Medical Association* (Zahn & Miller, October 8, 2003), "Although medical injuries are recognized as a major hazard, little is known about their impact." To evaluate this impact the researchers looked at extra days spent in the hospital, additional charges, and death rates from medical injuries. They concluded that costs resulting from injuries occurring during hospitalization ranged from no additional costs for obstetric trauma with minor repair to excess charges as high as $58,000 for serious infections occurring after an operation. Likewise, additional days spent in the hospital ranged from none for newborn trauma up to 11 days for operative infection. The researchers concluded that the impact of such injury is highly variable; however, injuries incurred during hospitalization pose a significant safety threat to patients and incur a large financial impact on society.[10]

Error Defined

The Institute of Medicine defines an error as "a failure of a planned action to be completed as intended or the use of the wrong plan to achieve an aim." The first term describes the error in Jesica's case. The IOM goes on to describe various types of errors, including errors of omission and errors of commission.[11] An error of omission is something that was supposed to happen but did not. An example of this would be a missed dosage of medication. An error of commission means a patient gets something that he or she was not supposed to receive. Jesica suffered from an error of commission; she received a heart and lung of an incompatible blood type.

If a patient needs a specific X-ray and the X-ray is performed on the wrong person, the person who misses the X-ray experiences an error of omission. The other patient experiences an error of commission because he or she undergoes a diagnostic test that was not intended for that person. Harm may not occur with either patient; however, if the person who does not get the X-ray has a small fracture or other key finding that is missed and goes untreated, then harm most likely will occur.

Tip

When undergoing any diagnostic test, ask what your test is for and why it is being done. Read the paperwork you are given to ensure that everything is correct. Speak up immediately if something seems questionable.

Error Reaching the Patient

The Institute of Medicine further defines[12] an active error as an error that occurs "at the level of the frontline operator and whose effects are felt almost immediately" and a latent error as an error "in . . . design, organization, training, or maintenance that lead[s] to operator errors and whose effects typically *lie dormant* in the systems for lengthy periods of time."

Causes of medical errors are diverse, but fundamentally they are rooted in system breakdowns. James Reason has done extensive work on the occurrence of accidents in aviation, space travel, and the nuclear industry, including the Three Mile Island nuclear accident and the explosion of the space shuttle *Challenger*.

Reason explains, "Active [sharp end] failures are the unsafe acts committed by people who are in direct contact with the patient or system.[13] Latent conditions [latent errors] are the inherent processes that lead to sharp end errors; this is where root causes exist."

A simple way to understand this concept is to think of a flowing river. Some errors—latent ones—develop "upstream." The active error is the point of impact in the river where the damage is clearly visible. In Jesica's case, the active end of the error was that Jesica received organs with incompatible blood. The latent conditions were multiple and primarily were system communication failures between the organ donor center and the hospital. Latent errors are not clearly visible and are inherent in many processes. It is only a matter of time until all of the wrong processes collide and an active error occurs.

Another illustration that describes the sequence of latent errors is called the Swiss cheese effect.[14] Multiple layers of protection surround a patient. Most of these layers have flaws or holes, like the holes in Swiss cheese, that can be penetrated. Given the correct circumstances, diverse ways of performing the same tasks, and enough time, an error can travel through the imperfections in the barriers and reach the patient.

In Jesica's case, because the ABO compatibility confirmation process had worked successfully many times before, the health professionals involved could not see the latent conditions in the process until all the barriers were breached, resulting in the significant medical error. It is critical that the public understand the complex processes that can lead to conditions of harm. They can then be alert during the early stages of a process to question areas of concern.

Tip

Early in the process of receiving hospital or health care services, make note of any small item that is out of place, and correct it immediately. A small item that is out of place may ultimately be part of a latent condition that can lead to an error.

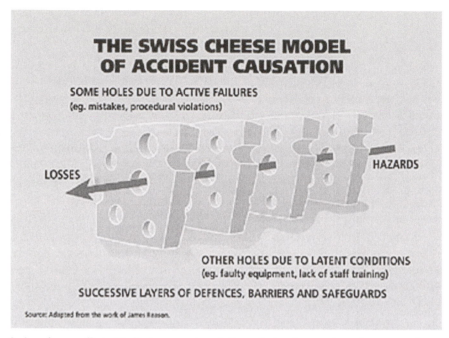

Swiss cheese effect. Medical errors travel through barriers and reach some patients. Illustration from James Reason.

Error Nomenclature

In health care, the nomenclature for defining medical errors is not standardized. The IOM has made the first attempt to clarify definitions. Standardization of error terminology will help the health care industry to better study errors, and this will help the public better understand the issues at hand.

The IOM defines an adverse event as "an injury caused by medical management, rather than the underlying condition of the patient."[15] An adverse event that is attributed to error is a preventable adverse event. The IOM found that 53 percent of adverse events are preventable.

Preventable or Not

One example of a preventable adverse event would be if a patient tells a hospital admitting clerk that he is allergic to penicillin, but the information never gets on the patient's chart. Following the patient's admission the doctor writes an order for a penicillin-related medicine. The nurse does not have the correct allergy information, nor does she check for allergies. The patient receives the penicillin-related medication and has a minor reaction. The health care team recognizes the reaction and quickly treats the patient. This reaction is an undesirable event and is a preventable adverse event because the health care professionals have an opportunity to catch the error before it reaches the patient.

In contrast, a nonpreventable adverse event occurs if a patient is not aware that he has an allergy to penicillin. Consequently, the patient tells the admitting clerk that he has no allergies. The penicillin-related medication is administered and the patient has a minor reaction. The health care team quickly treats the patient and no harm is done.

To keep preventable errors from reaching patients, the hospital should have a multisystem approach in place. It should improve its systems of communication, such as instituting a computer application that permanently records and transfers the patient's allergy status to any record that is used to treat the patient. For a simpler, less costly alternative, the hospital could use a special-colored wristband for patients with allergies. This would alert the nurse or clinician to the allergy before medications are administered.

Tip

Never assume that your doctor and other health care workers have communicated important facts about your care to each other. If you have an allergy to a medication, be sure that you repeat your allergy status to everyone giving you medicine.

LINDA

Unnecessary Radical Surgery Due to the Wrong Diagnosis

Linda McDougal, age 46, awoke from surgery with the anesthetic still lingering. She had been through a rough course. Two weeks earlier, Linda had been diagnosed with aggressive breast cancer. She and her husband made a harrowing, life-changing decision. Because she wanted to be around to see her three children grow up, she would undergo a bilateral mastectomy; removing both breasts was her best chance to beat the cancer and make a full recovery.

The next day, as Linda continued her postsurgical recovery, her surgeon came into her room and said, "I have bad news for you. You never had cancer." At first, Linda thought the surgeon meant that they got all the cancer during surgery and that would be good news. But when Linda asked her surgeon to clarify, she was told, "There was a mix-up in the lab."

Apparently, Linda's biopsy slides and paperwork were on the same tray as those of a patient with the aggressive cancer. The pathologist had mixed up the tests. Linda's breast tissue had been normal.[16]
How could such an error happen?

Given the Right Circumstances

Single errors such as those that Jesica, Ben, and Linda experienced appear to be isolated, but these errors are usually a combination of factors that converge into disaster. It would be easy to blame the nurses or doctors for these errors, but in each of these cases several dynamics collided that caused injury and death. If systems are not redesigned to be safer, then different doctors and nurses can still make similar errors today.

SHARON

Permanent Injury from Medication Error

In Minnesota, Sharon and James Williams were both established businesspeople and attorneys whose work took them traveling throughout Europe and Asia. Their marriage had produced two beautiful children.

Sharon had a history of painful uterine cysts and underwent surgery for a routine hysterectomy.

James said, "After surgery, when I saw her, I knew it was bad. She was jumping and twitching and her eyes were rolling all over the place." Sharon was in a coma. James later discovered that Sharon had been given an overdose of morphine in the recovery room after her surgery, and she stopped breathing. Sharon incurred irreversible brain damage and remains in a coma to this day.[17]

Medication Errors

Medical errors are significant, and a key subset of these errors involve medication errors, as evidenced by the cases of Ben Kolb and Sharon Williams discussed earlier. The IOM states that 7,000 people die each year as a result of medication errors and many more are harmed.[18] Hospitals use thousands of medications daily, many of which are beneficial and save lives. On the other hand, the administering of medications is a complex system, with many interacting parts and handoffs. Medication errors can occur during any of the steps involved in processing a medication.

These steps include handwriting an order, transcribing the order to other papers, using abbreviations, writing complicated drug names that may have similar spellings, preparing medications that may come in packaging that is similar to that of other medications, and mixing of drugs. This detailed process is prone to errors that include misplacing decimal points, making spelling errors, mixing the wrong drugs, administering a drug to the wrong patient, giving a drug through the wrong route, administering the wrong amount of a drug, and giving a drug at the wrong time. Studies have shown that 40 percent of errors occur in the administration of drugs, 21 percent occur because of documentation issues, 17 percent occur during the dispensing of drugs, 11 percent during the prescribing, and the remaining errors occur in other steps of the medication process.[19] The rate of adverse drug events has been reported to be as high as 6.5 percent within hospitals.[20] Upward of 56 percent of adverse drug events are preventable.[21]

Death by Decimal Point

At a children's hospital, a nine-month-old girl died after a misplaced decimal point caused a nurse to administer a massive overdose of morphine. Instead of two 0.5-mg doses of morphine, the baby was given two doses of 5 mg each—10 times what the surgeon intended—two hours apart as she recovered from successful surgery. Four hours after the second dose, the baby stopped breathing and went into cardiac arrest.[22]

Tip

Ask about all your medicines—what they are for, how they are to be given (injection, pills, etc.), when you are supposed to receive them,

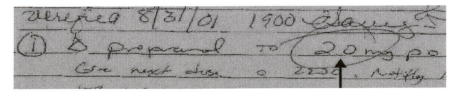

Dangerous abbreviations and dosage designations. Author unknown. *Source:* Retrieved September 2003 from http://patientsafety.ha.osd.mil.

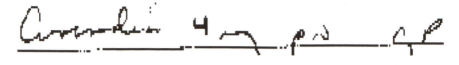

Coumadin, 4 milligrams by mouth (p.o.)? Coumadin is a drug that has been given to patients for years to help prevent blood clots. The order is actually for a new drug called Avandia, which is used to treat diabetes. You would not want to mistake these two medications. *Source:* Institute for Safe Medication Practices, www.smp.org.

whether there are any interactions between your other drugs or foods, and what side effects are possible.

Before taking any medication, especially if it looks unusual, ask your doctor and nurse about the medicine.

Tips

Health care professionals are required to check two forms of identification any time they administer medicines. Confirm that the clinician, usually a nurse, assures your identity. For example, they could ask you for your name and birth date.

For a family member who is under sedation or confused, confirm that the professional giving the medication confirms two forms of patient identifiers. Checking two separate identifiers on the wristband will accomplish this.

Early Warnings about the Spread of Infection

Long before the current practices of infection control were established, a brilliant Hungarian physician, Ignaz Semmelweis, who was teaching in Vienna began to see a correlation between germs and the spread of disease. In 1847, Dr. Semmelweis had a close friend, Jakob Kolletschka, who cut his finger while he was performing an autopsy. Kolletschka soon died of symptoms like those of puerperal fever (an infection that occurs after childbirth). Semmelweis watched as medical students went from the dissection laboratory to the delivery room without washing their hands. He attempted to implement a policy that students wash their hands between cases, but he was reprimanded by his supervisor and laughed at by his colleagues. It took another 15 years before Joseph Lister expanded on Semmelweis's hypothesis and began to use carbonic acid to kill germs. Semmelweis, whose theory continued to be rejected during his lifetime, died in a mental institution at the age of 47.

Health Care–Acquired Infections Today

Hospital-acquired infections are a prevalent problem in U.S. hospitals. Today, the practice of hand washing that Semmelweis first proposed is still fundamental to preventing the spread of infections. Hospitals carry a risk of infection by the very nature of their intradynamics: some people are admitted to the hospital with infections, antibiotic-resistant bacteria have been on the increase, and some patients are at risk for infections because of weak immune systems caused by illness. Also, the variety of health care workers who come in contact with patients presents many opportunities for bacteria transmission.

Resistance to Antibiotics

Widespread overuse of antibiotics has created mutations of bacteria that do not respond to common antibiotics. Two key types of resistant bacteria cause infection-related problems within hospitals:

1. Methicillin-resistant *Staphylococcus aureus* (MRSA)
2. Vancomycin-resistant enterococci (VRE)

Additional strains of resistant organisms are likely to cause increased problems in the future; however, the currently prevalent ones are discussed here. *Staphylococcus aureus (S. aureus)* is a common bacteria present on people's skin, in the nose, and in the environment. In most healthy people, *S. aureus* is not a problem. Within hospitals or other health care settings like nursing homes, however, *S. aureus* can cause serious problems, leading to surgical infections, bone infections, urinary tract infections, or pneumonia. Methicillin is a member of the penicillin family that has been effective in treating staph, but over the last several decades, the bacteria have become more resistant to both methicillin and vancomycin.[23]

MRSA and VRE infections cannot be successfully treated with methicillin and vancomycin, respectively. Specimen cultures are necessary to guide the physician as to the most appropriate treatment.

S. aureus can be spread from person to person through close contact with someone who is carrying the bacteria, especially by the hands or contaminated gloves. It can also be spread via other exposed items like clothing, medical tubing, towels, sheets, and medical supplies. It is not spread through the air. Proper hand washing is the single most important aspect in preventing the spread of these organisms.

Table 1.2
The Growth of Resistant Bacteria

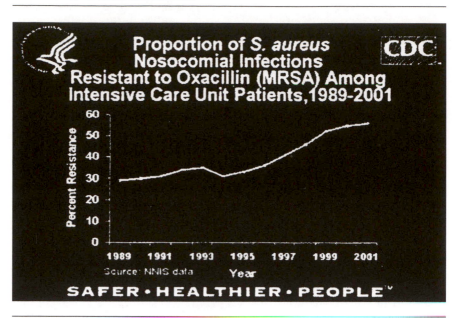

MRSA prevalence, as a proportion of health care–acquired *S. aureus* infections among ICU patients, 1989–2001. *Source:* Centers for Disease Control. (2003).

Some patients have large amounts of *S. aureus* colonized on their bodies. Colonization does not mean infection and may not cause any symptoms. Unless an infection is present a colonized person may not require treatment. Colonized people may develop an infection if they get a wound or become ill.

Health Care–Associated (Nosocomial) Infection

Health care–associated infection (HCAI), formally called nosocomial infection, refers to infection that occurs within a hospital, nursing home, or other health care facility and is not related to the original illness or condition. According to the Centers for Disease Control (CDC), the pervasiveness of HCAIs in U.S. hospitals is as high as two million occurrences a year and the cost is between $3.5 billion and $4.5 billion.[24, 25]

Not all, but many, HCAIs are preventable by excellent hand hygiene, rapid identification and isolation of infected patients, safe surgical practices, proper antibiotic use, and the correct use of protective gear such as gloves and wound dressings.

Surgical Site Infections

Infections involving the incision after surgery are known as surgical site infections. Different types of organisms, including those previously discussed, can cause surgical site infections. According to the CDC, the surgical site infection occurrence in hospitals is about 325,000 per year, costing hospitals approximately $1 billion.

Factors that contribute to these infections can be present during or after an operation. The most important measures in the prevention of surgical site infections are excellent surgical preparations and techniques as well as the appropriate use of presurgical antibiotics. The CDC provides extensive guidelines on the appropriate use and timing of antibiotics before surgery.

MR. E

Could Better Systems Have Prevented the Infection?

Mr. E, age 42, was scheduled for open-heart surgery at 1:00 P.M. His surgeon ordered an intravenous antibiotic to be given 30 minutes before the time of incision. The patient was prepared for the operation and at 12:20 P.M. was transported to the surgical hold area. The nurse in the hold area could not find the nurses' sheet where the floor nurse normally documented the antibiotic (the antibiotic was usually given on the floor). The sheet had been omitted from the patient's paper chart that came down with Mr. E.

The nurse in the hold area called the floor nurse, who was attending to another patient and unavailable. No one else on the unit could tell the hold area nurse if the antibiotic had been given. The hold area nurse did not want to administer the antibiotic twice. It was now 12:35 P.M. and the anesthesiologist, who was running late, called for the patient. As Mr. E was being moved out the door of the hold area, the floor nurse called the hold area nurse and told her that the antibiotic had not been given. The hold area nurse told the transport nurse to be sure to tell the anesthesiologist to administer the antibiotic. Mr. E was transported to the operating room and prepared for the incision. At 1:13 P.M., the surgical incision was made.

Later, as the transport nurse was moving another patient, she recalled that she forgot to tell the anesthesiologist to give the antibiotic. It was now 1:59 P.M. The anesthesiologist had assumed the medicine was already administered, and because the medication record from the floor was missing, no evidence existed to contradict that assumption. There was no antibiotic in the operating room, so it had to be delivered from the pharmacy. The antibiotic was finally given to Mr. E at 2:24 P.M., one hour and 54 minutes after it should have been administered.

Two days after the surgery, Mr. E developed a fever and redness at the incision site. The incision was cultured and showed an infection. Mr. E was started on an antibiotic, and he stayed in the hospital an additional two days. After he was discharged, his surgical incision became red and warm and started to drain fluid. He had to be readmitted to the hospital for another four days to treat the infection. The additional cost of treatment for his infection was $7,312. Mr. E, a self-employed painter, did not have health insurance and had to pay the additional cost out of his own pocket.

The use of paper charts, reliance on memory, and fragmented communication systems all contributed to the delay of Mr. E's antibiotic administration. Perhaps if Mr. E had been given the information regarding the need for a presurgery antibiotic, he may have been helpful in reminding the health professionals that he had not received the medication. Yet, improved systems need to be implemented so that no one factor that is excluded will lead to this error of omission.

Awareness about Infection

The consumer should be on the alert for the risk of acquiring an infection when hospitalized. Using excellent hand hygiene; being informed about presurgery antibiotics and the administration time; taking good care of intravenous lines, catheters for urine elimination, and drainage tubes; getting tubes and catheters out as soon as possible; and keeping surgical incision dressings clean and dry can all help to prevent a hospital infection.

Tips

When having surgery, talk to your surgeon before your operation. Ask what antibiotics you need and what time you need them. Make sure your doctor prints the name and time. Take this paper with you to the hospital and show the anesthesiologist and each of the nurses caring for you before the surgery.

If you have an incision from a procedure or surgery, strictly follow the instructions that you have been given.

Catheters are susceptible to infection. Work with your health care providers to remove any type of catheter as soon as possible.

Work with your health care team to get rid of all types of intravenous (IV) lines as soon as possible.

Infections are so prevalent within hospitals that the CDC is working aggressively with health care organizations, researchers, and hospital infection-control programs to prevent and reduce infections.

The CDC has targeted a 50 percent reduction in hospital infections over the next five years and asks for public comment on many of its projects.

Tips

For more information on the CDC and its work on the reduction of infections, log on to www.CDC.gov/drugresistance.

Ask the clinicians and health care workers taking care of you to wash their hands any time they will have direct contact with you.

If you are in the hospital, wash your hands frequently and thoroughly. Wash your hands before meals and after using the restroom.

If you are unable to get out of bed, ask the nurse or aide taking care of you to give you an antiseptic hand rub. Most hospitals provide these for bedridden patients who cannot go to the sink.

When you wash your hands, wash for as long as it takes you to sing the song "Yankee Doodle Dandy"; this is a great tip for children. Otherwise, wash your hands briskly for 15 to 30 seconds.

ALEXIS AND HER MOM

Two Medical Errors

In March 1999, Alexis Masiello was born with several birth defects. Now two years old, she had undergone multiple surgeries and had spent her entire life in a Massachusetts hospital. She had been fed through a tube and was dependent on a breathing tube as well.

Finally, little Alexis was going home. Her parents were very excited. They had prepared the house, and her father was going to be a stay-at-home dad. One night, several days before Alexis was to be discharged, a child-care worker noticed warning lights on the monitor in Alexis's room. Alexis's breathing tube had become disconnected. No one knew how long it had been that way. Although the hospital team tried to revive the toddler, she was unresponsive and died two days later.

Alexis's mom, Michelle, felt lost without Alexis and became severely depressed. One night, out of utter despair, Michelle took an overdose of pills and was rushed to the hospital. The medications she took made Michelle act wild; at the hospital she was given something to calm her, but at first it did not work. The staff had to put Michelle in restraints. While in restraints and left unattended, Michelle choked on the powderlike medicine she had been given to counteract the overdose. Michelle could not get out of the restraints and was unable to breathe.

The staff found Michelle unresponsive and tried to resuscitate her. She slipped into a coma and died 10 days later. Michelle died exactly nine months, to the day, after she lost Alexis.[26]

Restraint-Related Injuries and Death

The Joint Commission on Accreditation of Healthcare Organizations reports that 4.7 percent of voluntarily reported medical injuries and deaths are caused from restraints.[27] In 40 percent of the restraint deaths, the patient chokes and is unable to get free. The top three root causes for restraint injuries and deaths are inadequate training, poor communication, and inadequate patient assessment, all of which can be solved through better system designs.

The intent of using restraints is to help protect patients from harming themselves or others. Restraints are generally used as a last resort; yet their use is not uncommon in hospitals. Vest-type restraints are often used with elderly patients to prevent them from falling out of bed. Occasionally, restraints can be forceful, such as leather straps to hold violent patients trying to hurt themselves or others. State regulations are stringent for the use of restraints, but accidents still occur and caution must be used if a patient or family member is placed in any form of restraint.

Tips

If you have a family member who needs restraints, work with the health care team to determine if there are less restrictive ways to keep that family member safe. Often, confusion in a patient leads to the need for restraints. There may be other alternatives to protect the family member, such as the following:

> If you have a family member in the hospital who is confused or may be taking multiple medications that can cause confusion, ask that the patient be put on fall precautions. Fall precautions can include signs stating risk for fall, closer staff monitoring, and the removal of obstacles.

> Ask the staff to move a confused family member closer to the nurses' station. This move may be helpful, but remember that a patient care unit is a very busy place; proximity to the nurses' station is no guarantee that the family member will be constantly watched.

> If you have a family member who needs constant monitoring, talk to your nurse about obtaining a sitter. Generally, outside services provide sitters for a fee.

MRS. T

A Preventable Fall

Mrs. T, age 84, was in the hospital for treatment of an abnormal heart-beat. She was taking several heart medicines, and because she suffered from depression, she was on an antidepressive medication as well. Mrs. T seemed alert and understood the tests she was going to need; however, she was extremely nervous about being in the hospital.

During the evening, the primary doctor taking care of Mrs. T ordered an antianxiety drug to help calm her nervousness. Mrs. T was given the medicine, but the administration of the drug was not immediately recorded on the paper drug record. The nurse caring for Mrs. T had several other patients to care for as well.

Within an hour of administration of the antianxiety drug, Mrs. T's cardiologist came to see her. Mrs. T complained to her cardiologist about her nervousness, stating that she can never sleep when she is in the hospital because of all the noise. Her cardiologist ordered a medicine to help her sleep. Another nurse, who was covering for Mrs. T's nurse during a dinner break, administered the sleeping pill.

During the night, Mrs. T attempted to get out of bed to use the bathroom, became dizzy, and fell to the floor. The nurse's aide found Mrs. T on the floor, complaining of pain in both hips. The staff rushed her to X-ray. She had fractured both hips.

Some falls do not result in injuries, whereas others result in bruising, laceration, dislocation, fracture, and occasionally death. What happened to Mrs. T was the result of a combination of factors. She suffered from an abnormal heartbeat, which can aggravate dizziness. The night of her fall, she received an antidepressive medication, an antianxiety medication, and a sleeping medication. She was elderly, nervous, and in a strange environment. This combination of factors, perpetuated by a paper-reliant chart and vulnerable communication systems, made her highly susceptible to a preventable medical error, in this case, a fall.

The prevalence of falls within hospitals is hard to track in that there are no standard definitions or national databases to mandate reporting of patient falls. Of voluntary reportable events resulting in either serious injuries or death, 4.8 percent are falls.[28] Research shows that up to 70 percent of falls occur in patients over 68 years old. Falls are a common adverse event within hospitals, but many of them are preventable with appropriate communication and preventive system designs that help to identify patients at high risk of falling. Numerous hospitals study falls and attempt to make improvements in their reduction.

Even so, fall screening and prevention happen only sporadically, and incidents like Mrs. T's continue to occur within hospitals.

The Cost of Harm

The cost of medical errors, in terms of loss of life and harm to patients, is tremendous. The monetary cost of medical errors is also extraordinary. The Institute of Medicine states that the cost of medical errors is between $17 billion and $29 billion annually.[29] Half these costs are the result of direct health care, including additional days in the hospital, repeated surgeries, increased medications, and the treatment of complications. The other half are indirect costs such as lost income, lost productivity, and disability.

A study published in July 2002 by the Midwest Business Group on Health (MBGH), in conjunction with the Juran Institute in Chicago, substantiated the cost of poor-quality health care. For health plan members, MBGH reported that the increased cost for substandard quality of care is between $1,700 and $2,000 per employee.[30] One of the researchers, Joseph De Feo, found that $1,350 of the expenditure represented direct costs for providing services and the remaining portion represented indirect health care costs. De Feo stated, "A business cannot hope to thrive in the world markets while carrying this magnitude of unnecessary economic burden." The report identified that overuse, underuse, misuse, waste, and inefficiency were causes for these increased expenditures, specifying that 30 cents of every dollar was spent on these factors. Misuse included the cost of medical errors. The group listed drug prescription errors as the highest culprit, followed by hospital-acquired infections, surgical errors, and medical equipment problems.[31]

The consumer must absorb these health care costs in the form of higher insurance premiums and co-pays as well as taxes that support government-funded programs such as Medicare and Medicaid.

Changing the Error Factor

The error factor in health care is significant. Many factors contribute to the errors and are primarily related to complex systems and their many interactions. The Institute of Medicine's report discussed the need to move away from blaming individuals and look at solutions that redesign systems and avoid such errors as those described in this chapter. Health care consumers should be acutely aware that medical errors occur within hospitals and other health care settings and that errors can indeed happen to them. Consumers must understand that they are an important component in helping to prevent medical errors. Reading information carefully, speaking up, learning preventive tips, and questioning anything that seems out of place are the important first steps that a person can take to avert medical harm.

Health care professionals are also aware of risks that exist in hospitals and other settings, and they are working hard to redesign safer systems. Nevertheless, because of the complexity of health care, these changes will not come quickly. Physicians, pharmacists, nurses, and other health care professionals need the public's help to make these massive changes. Reducing medical errors will require a major culture change for health care, but that culture change will not happen effectively without the cooperation of the people whom health care was designed to serve—the patients. *Our key human error is that safer health systems are not being redesigned quickly enough to prevent tragic medical errors.*

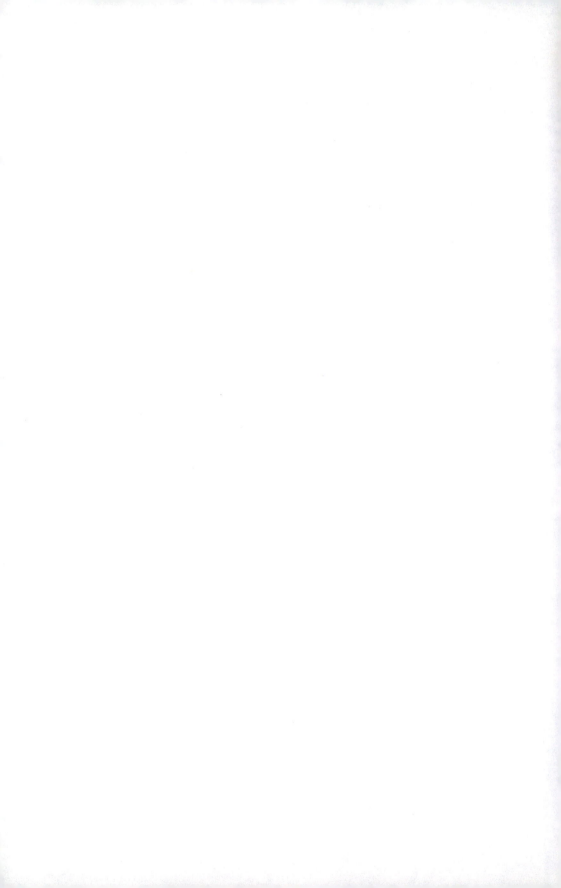

CHAPTER 2

COMMUNICATION VULNERABILITIES

And he goes through life, his mouth open, and his mind closed.

—Oscar Wilde

PAT

Missing Critical Information

In 1999, Pat Sheridan and his wife, Susan, lived in Boise, Idaho, with their son, Cal. Pat received terrible news that he had a tumor on his cervical spine. He was referred to one of the best neurosurgeons in the country. Pat and Susan traveled to Arizona so that Pat could have the tumor removed. After the surgery, they were relieved to hear that the tumor was benign; it was identified as a Schwannoma tumor, a slow-growing tumor that results from an overgrowth of the normal Schwann cells that surround nerve fibers in the body.

Six months later, to the couple's shock and dismay, a larger, more invasive tumor was found to be growing on Pat's spinal cord. This time the tumor was malignant. Pat again traveled out of state to undergo months of intensive chemotherapy. He participated in oncology clinical trials in hopes of curtailing the tumor's growth. Pat and Susan assumed that the first tumor had regrown and had become malignant.

As Pat and Susan started to look for answers, they discovered that the pathology report from the first surgery had shown a malignancy. Twenty-

two days after the initial surgery Pat's pathology report was placed in his medical record in Arizona. The malignancy results were never communicated to the neurosurgeon, and hence the surgeon did not communicate these results back to Pat in Idaho.[1]

Pat died in 2002, after undergoing seven surgeries to try to stave off the cancer in his spine.

Communication Breakdown

Communication failures are a central factor in medical errors. According to an article in *Annals of Internal Medicine*, invasive procedures done on the wrong patients occur far more frequently than reported. The article reviews a case in which an invasive cardiac procedure was performed on the wrong patient, despite the patient's attempts to communicate that she was not scheduled for the procedure. The case included 17 errors, both active and latent. One of the key findings of the investigation that followed the incident showed that communication failures were central to the mistake:

> Perhaps the most striking feature of this case—one that will be familiar to all clinicians who have worked in large hospitals—is the frighteningly poor communication it exemplifies. Physicians failed to communicate with nurses, attendings failed to communicate with residents and fellows, staff from one unit failed to communicate with those from others, and no one listened carefully to the patient. Although no data exist to document how widespread communication failures are, they are probably endemic in large, complex academic medical centers.
>
> Nevertheless, we suspect that these physicians and nurses had become accustomed to poor communication and teamwork. A "culture of low expectations" developed, in which participants came to expect a norm of faulty and incomplete exchange of information. Nurses had probably observed many instances of patients' lacking information about planned procedures. . . . Similarly, residents may have grown accustomed to being unaware of all the tests or treatments ordered by attendings, and physicians may have often failed to fully inform nurses about treatment plans. The combined impact of these experiences probably led these conscientious professionals to discount the numerous warning signals present in this case. The culture of low expectations led each of them to conclude that these red flags signified not unusual, worrisome harbingers but rather mundane repetitions of the poor communication to which they had become inured.[2]

Communication Complacency

Complacency with regard to poor communication has become an increasing problem in hospitals. Some doctors and health care professionals have grown to expect poor communication as the norm. Younger physicians and health care professionals have little knowledge of the time when better-functioning communication systems existed. Often, older physicians or nurses will say, "Hospitals aren't like they used to be; patients aren't getting the care they used to get." Communication systems have become overwhelmingly complex, to the point where younger health care professionals are learning to function within these flawed environments. Some older health care professionals are overwhelmed by the flawed systems but struggle with feasible solutions.

Tip

If a discrepancy exists in any action involving your care, speak up. If the person caring for you will not listen, find another health care professional and let him or her know there is a discrepancy.

The following is a review of three cases that focus on communication in health care. The first case almost resulted in an error, but it was averted because the patient was alert to the details of her care. The second scenario proceeded through care successfully due to new information technology and good communication venues. The last case resulted in a costly error.

MRS. U'S X-RAY

A Near Miss from Convoluted Communications Systems

Mrs. U developed a cyst on her right shoulder and went to see her primary physician. The doctor was concerned and wrote a prescription sending her to the radiology department across the street for an X-ray. The doctor also handwrote a referral to an orthopedic surgeon.

Before Mrs. U went for the X-ray, the primary doctor's nurse had to get an HMO authorization for both the orthopedic surgeon and the X-ray. Mrs. U knew an orthopedic surgeon who was outside the primary doctor's catchment area but was still part of the HMO plan. The office staff had never referred a patient to this orthopedic surgeon before, so the nurse also had to find this surgeon's contact information in order to complete the referral. The nurse and two members of the office staff made several phone calls to get the surgeon's

Handwritten prescription for an X-ray.

information. By the time the nurse had what she needed, there were two new patients in the waiting room and the nurse was feeling rushed.

The nurse completed the orthopedic surgeon's referral. She had difficulty reading the doctor's handwritten prescription for the X-ray. Since she was usually good at interpreting the doctor's writing, she attempted to decipher it without interrupting the doctor, who was now with another patient. She read it as "complete left shoulder X-ray." She transcribed the prescription to a handwritten X-ray order form.

The nurse gave the X-ray order and referral to Mrs. U, who took the paperwork across the street to the radiology department. Even though Mrs. U had previously been seen at this health care organization's other radiology departments, she was still required to complete new patient information forms. Mrs. U gave the clerk her demographic information. The process took 15 minutes. Mrs. U was given another form. She proceeded upstairs to the radiology area, handed the X-ray order form to the receptionist, and waited one hour. Finally Mrs. U was taken in for the X-ray.

As the technician began the X-ray of the left shoulder, Mrs. U stated, "It is my right shoulder," and pointed at the cyst. The technician apologized and asked the receptionist to change the paperwork. The receptionist redid the paperwork to state "right shoulder X-ray." The technician again began the X-ray.

Mrs. U then recalled that the doctor had said something about bilateral shoulder X-rays for a comparison and to check for other cysts. Mrs. U mentioned this to the technician, who again told the receptionist to correct the paperwork to "bilateral shoulder X-rays." The X-rays were completed.

Although this was only a simple diagnostic test, multiple opportunities for communication breakdowns existed in this scenario. Mrs. U's X-ray involved 19 handoffs, and each step allowed for an error to occur.

Let's evaluate this process. First, eight people were involved in this test:

1. The primary doctor
2. The primary doctor's nurse

3. The two office staff members who had to find the surgeon's information
4. The radiology department admitting clerk
5. The radiology department receptionist
6. The X-ray technician
7. The patient

Eight pieces of paper were generated:

1. The primary doctor's X-ray prescription
2. The primary doctor's referral prescription for the orthopedic surgeon
3. The HMO authorization form for the orthopedic surgeon
4. The nurse's order form for the X-ray (transcribed from the primary doctor's prescription)
5. The admitting paper
6. The first work order from the admitting clerk
7. The second work order
8. The final, and correct, work order

Outlined here are the communication vulnerabilities:

1. The primary doctor handwrote two prescriptions.

   Handwriting is open to multiple documentation errors and interpretations.

2. The doctor handed the two prescriptions to the nurse.

   No verbal confirmation of the correct side for the X-ray occurred between the doctor and the nurse; the conversation focused on finding the orthopedic surgeon's contact information.

3. The nurse transcribed the two prescriptions to the referral forms.

   Again, this transcribing process is open to documentation and interpretation errors.

   No verification occurred between the patient and the nurse.

   Although Mrs. U was standing next to the nurse, the nurse did not ask Mrs. U to confirm the side for the X-ray, and Mrs. U could not see what the nurse was writing.

4. The nurse handed the two new forms to the patient.

   The patient did not review the paperwork. Mrs. U assumed it was correct.

5. The patient handed the X-ray form to the radiology admitting clerk.

Neither the clerk nor the patient mentioned the details of the test, especially the side for the X-ray.

6. The admitting clerk created a new demographic form and the first work order.

   The frustration of having to reenter her demographic information was a distraction for the patient, and she did not focus on the X-ray.

7. The clerk handed the new work order to the patient and the patient signed the demographic/financial sheet.

   The clerk did not verify with the patient the correct side and site as it appeared on the new work order.

8. The patient took the work order to the radiology receptionist.

   The receptionist did not confirm with the patient the correct side for the X-ray.

9. The receptionist handed the work order to the X-ray technician.

10. The technician began to prepare for the left shoulder X-ray.

    The technician did not confirm with the patient the correct side or site for the X-ray.

11. The patient corrected the technician.

12. The technician handed the paperwork back to the receptionist.

    The technician did not question the lack of an order for comparison X-rays, although he mentioned later that he thought about it at the time because bilateral X-rays are often done in this type of case.

13. The receptionist changed the paperwork.

    The receptionist did not call the primary doctor to confirm the correct side and site for the X-ray.

14. The receptionist handed the order back to the technician.

15. The patient again corrected the technician.

16. The technician handed the paperwork back to the receptionist.

    Throughout this whole process, no health care worker called the doctor's office or asked the patient to confirm the correct side for the X-ray.

17. The receptionist corrected the work order again.

18. The receptionist handed the paperwork back to the technician.

19. The correct X-ray was done.

Duplicate processes and delays included creating eight pieces of paper, reentering the patient's demographic information, rewriting the order multiple times, and beginning the X-ray procedure three times. The error occurred originally when the nurse misread the prescription and transcribed the incorrect side for the X-ray.

There are two ways that this error might have been avoided:

1. Using an electronic medical record would allow each party involved in a patient's care, such as the nurse, office workers, and radiology departments, to receive an order as soon as the doctor enters it. Although these electronic systems are expensive, any cost-benefit analysis must consider the expenses incurred when employees continually repeat steps, introducing many opportunities for errors.

2. A less expensive solution would be for the doctor to hand print the prescription and allow the patient to take it with him or her to the admitting department. This would reduce the transcription process to one step, from the printed order to the work order.

Handwriting misinterpretations are central to multiple medical errors. More about handwriting will be discussed in later chapters.

Tip

When your paperwork is transcribed to another piece of paper, always read the new paper carefully to confirm that the information is the same as on the original.

Can you read the order? Tegretol or Tequin? Both come in 400-mg strengths. *Source:* Institute for Safe Medication Practices, retrieved 7 March 2003 from Medication Safety Alert, ismp.org.

Good Communication Systems Do Exist

The second scenario demonstrates improved communication venues that utilize less duplication and rely more heavily on technology solutions to reduce errors.

MRS. U'S MRI

One week later, the orthopedic surgeon saw Mrs. U and evaluated the X-rays (Mrs. U had hand carried the X-rays to the surgeon's office). He identified the cyst as an abnormal bone structure, possibly from an old injury, and he ordered an MRI electronically through his office online computer system.

The next day Mrs. U arrived at a different radiology department, but one that was still part of the same health care system. A file and wristband with Mrs. U's information was completed and waiting for her when she arrived. The receptionist confirmed Mrs. U's identity and asked to see her insurance card to confirm that nothing had changed. Mrs. U waited 10 minutes. The MRI transporter called Mrs. U and introduced himself as Matt. Mrs. U traveled with Matt to the MRI area.

The MRI technician and Mrs. U discovered that they knew each other, but the technician still insisted on checking her wristband. The technician confirmed the correct side and site with Mrs. U and explained the procedure. Mrs. U underwent the MRI successfully. The technician told Mrs. U that the radiology film reports were part of an electronic system and that the surgeon would instantly see an electronic result on his computer. As a backup, the technician made a copy of the films and gave them to Mrs. U. He told her to take the films with her to the surgeon's office. Matt took Mrs. U back to the waiting room.

What are the differences in communication between these two diagnostic tests? With Mrs. U's second experience a number of processes were streamlined and more efficient.

First, fewer people were involved in the process:

1. The receptionist
2. The transporter
3. The MRI technician
4. The patient

Three forms of communication were utilized in the process:

1. The electronic order from the orthopedic surgeon's office
2. The MRI work order
3. The patient's previously registered demographic sheet
4. The electronic results

There were seven handoffs in this process, compared to 19 in Mrs. U's visit to the first radiology facility:

1. The surgeon's office sent an electronic order for the MRI to the radiology department before the patient arrived.

2. The radiology department used an electronic registration system and noted that the patient had been at the center before.

   Because the surgeon's order was typed it was clear to read and confirmation of the correct shoulder could be done, eliminating interpretation errors that can occur with handwritten orders.

3. The patient arrived and the receptionist reconfirmed the patient's information for accuracy, providing a double-check system.

4. The patient was called by name and escorted to the MRI area.

5. The MRI technician reconfirmed the patient identity as well as the side and site for the procedure.

6. The test was completed.

7. The patient was given a copy of the films.

One might argue that the MRI was planned and Mrs. U's first X-ray was not. Even so, the unplanned X-ray was a simple diagnostic test. Unplanned events and interruptions are normal in health care because people's needs are ever changing, and a system should be able to handle such events efficiently. In a fragmented communication system the inability to handle even simple unplanned tests creates the opportunity for errors. Improved processes, technology, and communication venues can be designed to allow for interruptions without increasing the probability of medical errors.

Tips

You can check out (as a loan) your own X-ray or imaging studies from your radiology center.

Always carry your own X-rays or imaging studies with you when you are referred to a specialist.

When signing out studies from your radiology department, check the films to make sure they are correct. Sometimes films are placed in the wrong film jackets.

If you have had multiple X-rays or imaging studies taken at the same facility, check the film jacket to ensure that it contains the right test performed on the right day. Look at the corner of the actual film, where your name, the date, and the type of test will be printed.

Wear minimal or no jewelry or metal when having an X-ray or imaging study, as you will be asked to remove such items so they will not be seen on the films. Although your personal items are generally secured during your test, they can be lost or stolen.

Multilayered Communication

Good communication is central to any successful process. Few hospitals have centralized electronic medical records; most hospitals have multiple stand-alone computer systems. This can result in a lack of coordination among departments: surgical scheduling may differ from that in the cardiac cath lab, the laboratory program may not interface with radiology, or outpatient registration may be isolated from other departmental registrations.

How did hospitals end up with these multilayered communication systems? Over time, hospitals have attempted to keep up with current information technology. Cost has always been an issue, however. Large, integrated technology solutions and computer systems are expensive, ranging in the millions of dollars. Hospitals generally buy or upgrade isolated technologies that may solve select individual department needs, but they do not solve the larger communication issues. Sometimes, the layering of isolated systems causes more dangers; the systems may not effectively communicate with each other, building latent conditions into the communication structure that may not be visible until an active error occurs. In hindsight, the active error clarifies the risk that had lain dormant.

In implementing isolated solutions in an attempt to control costs, hospitals may be spending far more on the duplication of time, services, resources, and paying for medical errors than they would pay by investing in long-term, integrated technology solutions.

MRS. HOFFMANN

Hearing the Patient

Mrs. Hoffmann, an immigrant from Germany, was scheduled for a cardiac angioplasty and stent placement to open her two partially blocked coronary arteries. Mrs. Hoffmann and her son entered a busy New York hospital. The admitting nurse took a medical history. Mrs. Hoffmann was in the very early stages of Alzheimer's but was still able to function independently with her medications. She also suffered from arthritis and mild depression in addition to her heart problems. Mrs. Hoffmann did not have a written list of her medicines, but she was able to tell the nurse what she was currently taking: Reminyl, vitamin E, Celebrex, Monopril, aspirin, and a nitroglycerin patch. The nurse asked her son to confirm the medications and he said, "I'm pretty sure what Mom said is correct. It sounds like the medicines that I pick up at the pharmacy." The nurse wrote the medicines as follows:

Remeron, vitamin E, Celebrex, Monopril, aspirin, nitro patch

Mrs. Hoffmann was admitted to the cardiac unit and was scheduled for a 3:00 P.M. procedure. The cardiologist had written orders for Mrs. Hoffmann's procedure and called the primary physician to confirm her medicines. The primary physician was out of town and the doctor covering for his colleague's patients was at another hospital attending to an emergency. He did not have access to Mrs. Hoffmann's medications.

By this time, Mrs. Hoffmann's cardiologist had two new emergency heart patients who had arrived downstairs in the emergency room. Since Mrs. Hoffmann's son had confirmed the medications, the cardiologist added to the written order the medications that Mrs. Hoffmann had given to the admitting nurse.

Mrs. Hoffmann's procedure was delayed because the cardiologist had to perform emergency angioplasty procedures on both emergency room patients. The doctor rescheduled Mrs. Hoffmann to have her angioplasty the next morning.

That evening, Mrs. Hoffmann was given her medications. When the nurse handed Mrs. Hoffmann the Remeron, Mrs. Hoffmann said, "This pill is different than the pill I take at home." The nurse assumed that the pharmacy had stocked a generic brand of pills and explained this to Mrs. Hoffmann. The nurse asked, "What is the medicine you take at home?" Mrs. Hoffmann said, "Reminyl," but because of her heavy German accent, the nurse was sure Mrs. Hoffman said Remeron. Remeron had been used to treat depression for several years and the nurse was used to administering it. At the time, Reminyl was a new medicine that had recently been approved for use in Alzheimer's patients, and the nurse was not familiar with it. The nurse rechecked the order. The order said Remeron, so she administered the medication, although Mrs. Hoffmann again said, "This looks different."

The next day, Mrs. Hoffmann woke up early in the morning with some chest pressure. She called the nurse and said, "This is the pressure I get in my chest when my heart is bothering me."

The physician ordered an ECG and cardiac blood tests. Mrs. Hoffmann was experiencing some abnormalities in her heart rhythm and the cardiologist wanted to treat her first with some medicines before doing the angioplasty. She was treated on the floor for two days.

One evening, Mrs. Hoffmann's son was visiting when a different nurse brought in the Remeron. The son noted that the medication looked different from what his mother took at home. He mentioned that it was important for his mother to have the right medicine because of her Alzheimer's. The nurse checked the order and said that this was what the doctor ordered, and she administered the medication.

On the fourth day of Mrs. Hoffmann's hospitalization, she was again scheduled for her heart procedure. Mrs. Hoffman was becoming confused and could not remember why she was in the hospital. The nurses continually reassured Mrs. Hoffmann and reminded her that she was having an angioplasty. Mrs. Hoffmann was taken in for the cardiac procedure.

When the procedure was completed, Mrs. Hoffmann became combative, flinging her body wildly. She attempted to get up off the procedure table. The staff tried to restrain her and called an emergency restraint code. Mrs. Hoffmann was very strong, and in all of the commotion, she dislodged the large catheter in her groin and began to bleed profusely. The cardiac team was finally able to restrain her; the cardiologist repositioned the catheter and repaired the site, and the bleeding stopped.

After the incident, the cardiologist contacted the primary care physician's office to inform the primary physician of Mrs. Hoffmann's status. She was puzzled by Mrs. Hoffmann's behavior and thought the Alzheimer's was progressing more readily than first determined. The primary care physician told the cardiologist that she would increase the Reminyl. The cardiologist replied, "What Reminyl?"

Tips

When going to the hospital, bring along a neatly printed or typed list of all the medications you take, including vitamins, herbs, and supplements. Make sure you check the correct spelling of the items and write down the exact doses and times that you take the medicines.

At home, keep your medication list posted on your refrigerator with a magnet. Be sure that *all* the medicine names are spelled correctly. Write your doctor's name and phone number, dosages, and the times you take the medications on the list as well. In case of an emergency, paramedics can take the list to the hospital. Update this list regularly.

Inaccurate Communication Processes

Mrs. Hoffmann's experience is not an isolated event. Because of the inappropriate use of the medicines, Mrs. Hoffmann required three additional days in the cardiac unit, four days in a skilled nursing care unit, three additional medications, a transfusion of red blood cells, and minor surgery to repair her groin area. The additional cost for this treatment was $24,812.

A full investigation was completed. The conclusion was that multiple systems failed, although two systems were central to the medical error: first, the communication systems failed to record and transfer information about the patient's correct medications, and second, more importantly, no one listened to the patient and her family member when they expressed concern about the medications.

Hospitals and health care industries have not implemented communication systems with the intention of having them fail. But because so many isolated solutions are in place, the layering has resulted in communication vulnerabilities throughout.

Hearing the Patient Again

Health care professionals are taught to assess and listen to their patients. Nonetheless, the actual practice of listening has become diluted. Health care professionals have a broad base of knowledge and experience. Their knowledge and experience have no doubt helped many patients. Even so, the assumption that "we know what's best" may actually be dangerous if it supersedes the fundamental principle of listening to the patient. Patients often know a great deal about their illnesses, medicines, and treatments. When patients question the clinician, they should be heard and their ideas incorporated into care. In addition, to bring about the massive changes that the health care industry needs to accomplish, patients have to be the hub of safety improvements and significant reductions in medical errors.

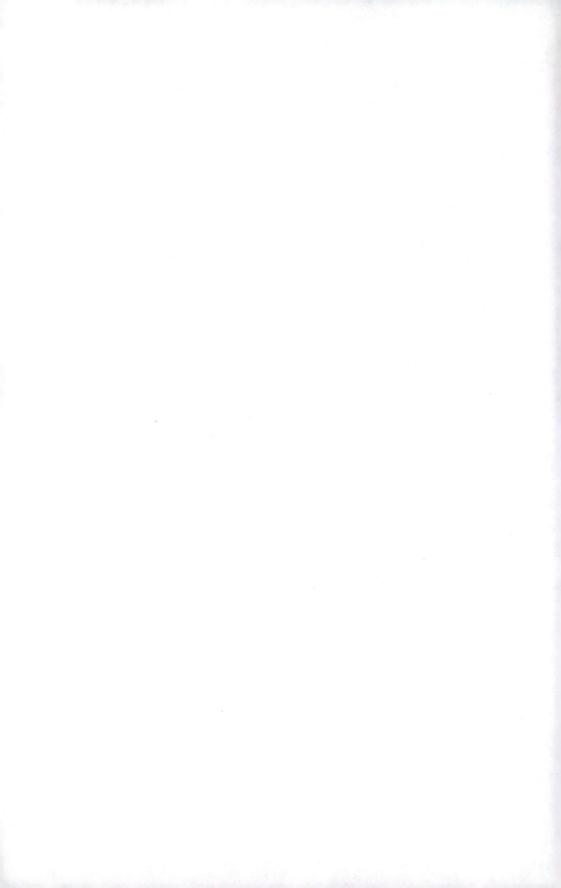

CHAPTER 3

WHY THE SILENCE?

"Sponge left in patient, massive infection develops."

Many hospital CEOs have been mortified to find such a headline leaping out at them from the front page of their local newspaper. Unfavorable articles about medical mishaps are upsetting and can paint a bad picture of the hospitals involved. Fear of public detection of medical errors is a significant issue for hospital leaders.

Truth be known, this type of headline is like an iceberg. Even in hospitals with a good reputation, errors that surface represent only a small portion of the actual adverse events that occur. The public knows little about these events. Hospital administrators do not, nor are they obligated to, report every medical injury or death that occurs within their facility. The discovery of any mishap by the local newspaper is usually the result of a disgruntled patient or happenstance.

How Far Has Health Care Come in Reducing Errors?

BETSY LEHMAN

Chemotherapy Overdose

In 1994, Betsy Lehman, age 39, a prominent health reporter for the Boston Globe, developed breast cancer. After completion of an intense course of chemotherapy at the Dana-Farber Cancer Institute, a world-renowned center for the treatment of cancer, she was scheduled for discharge.

David Warsh, a Globe *reporter, later wrote about the last day of Betsy's life.[1] That day Betsy felt as if something was wrong—very wrong. She phoned a friend and left a message: "I am feeling frightened, very upset. I don't know what is wrong, but something's wrong." It was almost as if a sense of doom overwhelmed her. An hour later, she was dead.[2] What had happened?*

Betsy had received a fourfold overdose of a potent chemotherapy drug intended to treat her cancer. She received 26 grams of the cancer-fighting agent over four days, though she was supposed to receive only 6.5 grams. Betsy died the day she was scheduled to go home to her husband and two children, three and seven years old. In a separate incident, not well publicized, another woman at the Dana-Farber institute received an overdose of chemotherapy during the same period as Betsy. She had to be rushed to the intensive care unit for treatment of drug toxicity. She survived.

Betsy's case received extensive national attention primarily because of her position with the Boston Globe. *A later investigation revealed a series of latent conditions and system design flaws that allowed for such a significant misinterpretation of the physician's order.*

Betsy's death caused a public outcry, and the Dana-Farber Institute made significant improvements to prevent this type of error from recurring. Nevertheless, nearly a decade later, people are still being harmed by medical errors related to chemotherapy and other toxic drugs.

- *In November 1997, in a New Jersey teaching hospital, a 10-month-old died after receiving 204 milligrams, instead of 20.4 milligrams, of cisplatin, a potent chemotherapy medication.[3]*

- *In the summer of 2002, at a Maryland hospital, a two-year-old boy lost his hearing after receiving an overdose of the chemotherapy drug Carboplatin. A health official stated, "It's clear their systems broke down. They miscalculated the amount of the drug, gave the wrong dose three days in a row, and we have a bad outcome."[4]*

- *In December 2003, a two-year-old girl who suffered from cancer died at the Johns Hopkins Children's Center in Baltimore of a potassium overdose. Her parents stated that their child died as a result of "a cascade of failures."[5]*

Since Betsy Lehman's death, progress has moved slowly toward preventing overdoses of chemotherapy and other toxic medications. Research published in the American Journal of Health-System Pharmacy *on medication-related deaths occurring between 1993 and 1998 found that chemotherapy errors were the second most common cause of death.[6]*

Tip

If you need to receive chemotherapy, learn everything you can about
the medication, including the correct dose, duration of treatment, side
effects, and how the drug will be administered and by whom.

Obstacles to Improvements in Safety

Why are the reductions in medical errors moving so slowly? The
obstacles encountered in making swift changes are complex. Health
care leaders recognize the severity of the problem and often make
small, incremental improvements in processes as errors occur.
However, most of these changes do not address the need for large-
scale system redesigns to substantially minimize latent conditions.

With each significant error, a hospital team internally investigates
the facts and immediate steps are taken to prevent recurrence. Yet it
is clear that larger system redesigns such as integrated computer systems, automated checks of medication administration, fail-safe medical equipment, and safer environments to prevent human error must
be implemented. On the other hand, these redesigns are expensive
and take time to implement. Additionally, research on patient safety
solutions is limited because many of the proposed safety solutions are
new and have not been well tested in actual patient environments.

Another reason for the slow change is that hospital tracking mechanisms for errors are convoluted and fragmented. The data collection, analysis, and reporting of injuries are not standardized, and the
data are often buried in an information quagmire. Current internal
data systems have limitations and are often considered subjective
since they are not controlled to the same extent as sound clinical
research data.

Incident Reports

Most hospitals track a form most commonly known as an incident
or occurrence report (see sample risk incident report at the end of
this chapter). Incident reports detail events such as medication
errors, surgical errors, unexpected patient deaths, patient falls, laboratory mishaps, blood reactions, X-ray issues, delays, mistaken
patient identities, near misses, and other patient adverse events. A
near miss has been defined as an error that almost reaches the patient
but is avoided before the patient is actually harmed. A near miss
might be as simple as almost giving an aspirin to the wrong patient

or as significant as nearly performing surgery on the wrong side or site.

Incident reports are not part of the patient record and are not shared with patients. The reports are protected from legal discovery and are generally not released outside of the hospital. Quality and risk management departments strictly control the flow of these forms within the hospital. Often many health care professionals and workers cannot tell you the full process for how error data are tracked. Employees and physicians complete incident reports. Depending on the specific hospital, staff and physicians may see trended results of the data, but there seems to be no standardized use across hospitals. Most hospitals have some version of these forms for internal quality tracking. Also, depending on the size of individual hospitals, anywhere from 30 to 300 incident reports are generated each month. Large health care systems with multiple facilities can track as many as 1,000 events each month. Keep in mind that not all incidents are adverse events; some may be as simple as a delayed response from a physician that does not result in harm.

Use of Incident Report Data

Hospitals use data from incident reports in various ways. The data may be trended by category; for example, delays in laboratory testing are grouped together and the laboratory manager reviews the trends and looks for common problems in order to make improvements. Some hospitals generate trend reports that are sent to department managers on a monthly or quarterly schedule. Other hospitals do not run trend reports but instead review incident reports on a case-by-case basis.

The incident report process can be overwhelming for a hospital. It takes a great deal of human resources to decipher reliable and valid trends; therefore, hospitals vary in their fiscal commitment to this process. Some hospitals still use handwritten incident reports, which are labor-intensive to read and interpret. As information databases improve, hospitals will most likely improve their ability to track alarming trends. Currently, such trends may be lost amid the volume of handwritten paperwork.

Some hospitals are beginning to move to partially or completely computer-based incident report tracking, which helps to better identify worrisome trends. Nonetheless, many electronic tracking systems are expensive, and an appropriate number of computers is not always available to the staff.

Tips

If an error occurs while you are in the hospital, even if it is minor, ask the person caring for you to complete an incident report. This can help the hospital look for similar errors so it can prevent a recurrence.

Quality or risk management departments in most hospitals track error data. Many of the hospital workers are unfamiliar with all of the errors and how the data are used. For information on error tracking at your hospital, call the quality or risk management department.

Doctors' use of incident report data varies widely. Some physician leaders may use the data to monitor trends and implement safety measures and clinical improvements. Other physicians feel that these incident reports lack relevant clinical data and hence do not rely on them for improvement. Incident reports or trended data are often included in physicians' credentialing profiles (credentialing profiles will be described in chapter 4).

Even though hospitals have policies describing the incident report process, the nomenclature of medical errors has not been standardized in U.S. hospitals and health organizations. Therefore, hospital staff may have subjective opinions about what constitutes a medical error or near miss. Minor or moderate events may not be viewed as mistakes, especially if the hospital worker does not recognize the incident as an error but rather as related to the patient's illness. At the active end of a less serious error, it is not always easy to evaluate the steps, especially the latent conditions, that led to an adverse event.

MRS. C

Hidden Error

Mrs. C, age 70, underwent a cardiac catheterization to determine if she had blocked coronary arteries. The contrast dye that was injected to make her arteries visible for the procedure was to be filtered and excreted from the body through the kidneys.

No kidney tests were done before her catheterization, and unknown to the doctor, Mrs. C had impaired kidney function. Following the procedure, Mrs. C became nauseated and unable to urinate. She could not properly excrete the contrast dye from her kidneys, and this caused a temporary decrease in her kidney function. She was admitted to the hospital for treatment.

The nurse taking care of Mrs. C did not link Mrs. C's kidney problems to her reaction to the contrast dye. Mrs. C's hospitalization may have been avoided if a kidney function blood test had been performed before her heart catheterization. The abnormal kidney results could have guided her cardiologist to use a diluted contrast dye or to lessen the amount of contrast dye used. The nurse caring for Mrs. C did not perceive or report this as an adverse event, yet this incident meets the definition of a preventable medical error.

Another hindrance to employees' completion of incident reports is the fear of blame or punishment. This concept will be explored more extensively in later chapters.

Tips

When undergoing a procedure using contrast dye, discuss with your doctor your risk of kidney problems. Older adults and people with diabetes and kidney disease need to be especially careful about their kidney function when receiving contrast dye.

Kidneys excrete the contrast dye used in radiology and other procedures. Discuss with your physician the risk of having contrast dye for any procedure.

Be aware of a possible allergic reaction to contrast dye. Incidents of allergic reaction to contrast dye have been reported as between 1 in 1,700 and 1 in 4,500.[7]

Silence

Given that hospitals track many incidents of near misses, patient harm, and deaths, why don't consumers know more about these errors? The main reason for the silence is that current laws protect error data from legal discovery and release to the public.

In 1986, with support from the medical community, Congress passed the federal Health Care Quality Improvement Act (HCQIA), which protects from legal discovery error data that fall under physician peer review. The act protects physician peer review committees and their activities from legal discovery. When adverse events occur within hospitals, the information and investigation about the errors are discussed in closed meetings with physicians and support staff. No outside people are allowed to attend. The discussions that take place at the meetings and the decisions the physicians make regarding the case are protected from legal discovery and public release. In other words, any incident reports or other documents cannot be released to attorneys or courts for review.

The Health Care Quality Improvement Act

Medical associations support the HCQIA because they maintain that physicians can best police or peer-review their cases when they do not fear legal retaliation. The act was built on the premise that doctors would not be forthright and open in their discussions, actions, and quality improvements in patient case reviews if medical malpractice attorneys could access the information. The intent is also to give state medical boards the authority to discipline physicians according to their own codes and regulations.

The legislation is described here:

The intent [of the act] is to improve the quality of health care by encouraging State licensing boards, hospitals and other health care entities, and professional societies to identify and discipline those who engage in unprofessional behavior; and to restrict the ability of incompetent physicians, dentists, and other health care practitioners to move from State to State without disclosure or discovery of previous medical malpractice payment and adverse action history. Adverse actions can involve licensure, clinical privileges, professional society membership, and exclusions from Medicare and Medicaid.[8]

In addition, legislation from the HCQIA protects data under peer review as outlined in the five intents listed here.

The Congress finds the following:

1. The increasing occurrence of medical malpractice and the need to improve the quality of medical care have become nationwide problems that warrant greater efforts than those that can be undertaken by any individual State.

2. There is a national need to restrict the ability of incompetent physicians to move from State to State without disclosure or discovery of the physician's previous damaging or incompetent performance.

3. This nationwide problem can be remedied through effective professional peer review.

4. The threat of private money damage liability under Federal laws, including treble damage liability under Federal antitrust law, unreasonably discourages physicians from participating in effective professional peer review.

5. There is an overriding national need to provide incentive and protection for physicians engaging in effective professional peer review.[9]

In reality, the legislative intent of the first and third items in the preceding list has not been accomplished. The truth is validated by the Institute of Medicine's report stating that upward of 98,000 people die each year from medical errors, a report that was released well after passage of the HCQIA of 1986. In addition, the current volume of medical malpractice litigation is evidence of the legislation's failure to achieve its intent. This subject will be discussed in chapter 10, "Beyond Medical Malpractice."

Looking for Bad Apples

The belief behind the HCQIA legislation is that incompetent or impaired physicians are the root cause of poor quality. This belief supports the practice of looking for the "bad apples," a concept that targets individual blame and is contrary to the concepts outlined in the IOM report. The bad apple belief states that if we rid the industry of the bad or incompetent players, our problems of patient harm will be solved.

In addition, the bad apple theory goes against the philosophy of renowned quality leaders such as J. Edwards Deming and Joseph Juran. Through their work they have clearly established that poor quality stems from process variation, not from a few bad apples. Deming stated, "Organizations should focus on bad processes, not bad people. Ninety-four percent of all errors are system errors, not employee errors."[10]

Fewer Ways to Do the Same Thing Right

Performance improvement builds on the principle that with greater variation—that is, numerous ways to accomplish the same goal—it is more likely that outcomes will be diverse and unpredictable. Process variation can be harmful when it comes to establishing patient safety practices. For example, in the case study involving Mr. E, the process allowed for various people to administer the antibiotic to surgical patients at various times. If it was always administered in the preop area by the prep nurse, then the variation and chance for error would be diminished.

The use of standard protocols and processes helps to diminish errors. Reducing variation is the basis for improving patient safety and ultimately helping to reduce errors in hospital processes. Although more research is needed, medical malpractice litigation may be reduced if improved systems are implemented that allow for the reduction of process variation in medical procedures. It is a simple concept—complete procedures consistently, with less variation, within sound, structured systems and significantly reduce the chances of errors.

Intents two, four, and five of the legislation appear to be more successful in provoking physicians to freely discuss cases and to make isolated quality improvements. These intents have also assisted in tracking some incompetent or impaired physicians. Nevertheless, overall hospital system designs have not been enhanced through these legislative mechanisms.

The National Practitioner Data Bank

It is important to recognize that some physicians are indeed incompetent, impaired, or both. After all, the 6 percent of errors remaining in J. Edwards Deming's equation are not attributable to systems. As a result of the HCQIA legislation, the National Practitioner Data Bank (NPDB), which is administered by the Department of Health and Human Services, was created.

The NPDB is described as

> an alert or flagging system intended to facilitate a comprehensive review of health care practitioners' professional credentials. The information contained in the NPDB is intended to direct discreet inquiry into, and scrutiny of, specific areas of a practitioner's licensure, professional society memberships, medical malpractice payment history, and record of clinical privileges. The information contained in the NPDB should be considered together with other relevant data in evaluating a practitioner's credentials; it is intended to augment, not replace, traditional forms of credentials review.

Among physicians, the validity of the NPDB is often questioned. There are concerns that the data are inaccurate and old. In addition, just because a physician has malpractice claims or settlements against him or her does not necessarily mean that the physician is a bad practitioner. Despite that some practitioners are impaired or incompetent, these few practitioners are not the root cause of most medical errors.

Tip

To learn more about the legislation behind the National Practitioner Data Bank, log on to the Web site, http://www.npdb-hipdb.com. Note: You cannot review individual physician information. Access to this information is limited to hospitals, state boards, and government agencies.

State-Sanctioned Protections

Another reason for silence regarding medical errors is that in many states, additional laws protect peer-review data from discovery by patients and attorneys. In California, the law that protects quality and peer-review data is called California Evidence Code 1157. Its key components are listed here:

> §1157—. . . Neither the proceedings nor the records of organized committees of medical staffs in hospitals, or of a peer review body . . . having the responsibility of evaluation and improvement of the quality of care rendered in the hospital, or for that peer review body . . . having the responsibility of evaluation and improvement of the quality of care, shall be subject to discovery.[11]

Approximately 75 percent of states have additional peer review laws, although the HCQIA federal sanction helps protect medical staff data in the states that do not have their own peer review codes or laws.

Attorney-Client Privilege

Another protection afforded to hospital incident reports and error data involves attorney-client privilege. The data used to track patient harm are held through hospitals' risk management and quality departments. Because hospitals and their risk management departments are often represented by attorneys, attorney-client privilege applies to the designated error data. This protection has been challenged at state levels and historically has been argued successfully in favor of the hospital. As long as an incident report is marked confidential, the information is protected. In the case of Sierra Vista Hospital versus Superior Court (1967, 248 Cal. App. 2d 359), the judge ruled that incident reports are protected under attorney-client privilege.

Challenges of Protection

Physician peer-review laws have been challenged in court on multiple occasions. The rulings have continued to favor confidentiality of the peer-review process within hospitals if the judge deems that physicians participating in peer reviews are acting in good faith to improve quality. Several bills have been proposed—and continue to be hotly debated—that would allow for greater access to medical

Figure 3.1
Risk Incident Report

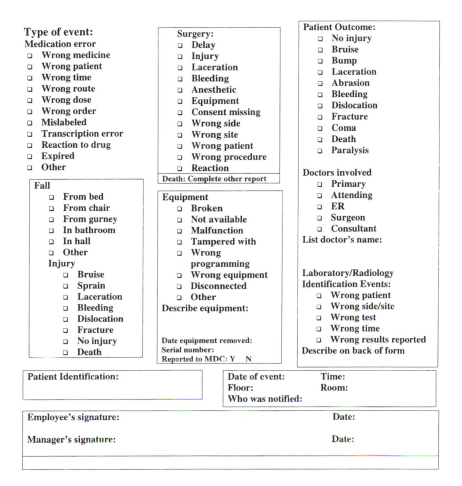

Description of event:

Describe patient's outcome and actions taken:

Type of event:
Medication error
- ❑ Wrong medicine
- ❑ Wrong patient
- ❑ Wrong time
- ❑ Wrong route
- ❑ Wrong dose
- ❑ Wrong order
- ❑ Mislabeled
- ❑ Transcription error
- ❑ Reaction to drug
- ❑ Expired
- ❑ Other

Fall
- ❑ From bed
- ❑ From chair
- ❑ From gurney
- ❑ In bathroom
- ❑ In hall
- ❑ Other

Injury
- ❑ Bruise
- ❑ Sprain
- ❑ Laceration
- ❑ Bleeding
- ❑ Dislocation
- ❑ Fracture
- ❑ No injury
- ❑ Death

Surgery:
- ❑ Delay
- ❑ Injury
- ❑ Laceration
- ❑ Bleeding
- ❑ Anesthetic
- ❑ Equipment
- ❑ Consent missing
- ❑ Wrong side
- ❑ Wrong site
- ❑ Wrong patient
- ❑ Wrong procedure
- ❑ Reaction

Death: Complete other report

Equipment
- ❑ Broken
- ❑ Not available
- ❑ Malfunction
- ❑ Tampered with
- ❑ Wrong programming
- ❑ Wrong equipment
- ❑ Disconnected
- ❑ Other

Describe equipment:

Date equipment removed:
Serial number:
Reported to MDC: Y   N

Patient Outcome:
- ❑ No injury
- ❑ Bruise
- ❑ Bump
- ❑ Laceration
- ❑ Abrasion
- ❑ Bleeding
- ❑ Dislocation
- ❑ Fracture
- ❑ Coma
- ❑ Death
- ❑ Paralysis

Doctors involved
- ❑ Primary
- ❑ Attending
- ❑ ER
- ❑ Surgeon
- ❑ Consultant
List doctor's name:

Laboratory/Radiology
Identification Events:
- ❑ Wrong patient
- ❑ Wrong side/site
- ❑ Wrong test
- ❑ Wrong time
- ❑ Wrong results reported
Describe on back of form

Patient Identification:

Date of event: Time:
Floor: Room:
Who was notified:

Employee's signature: Date:

Manager's signature: Date:

review board hearings and physician peer reviews. Generally, the courts deny release of physician peer-review cases or trends on physicians. Both peer-review and attorney-client privilege protections are powerful laws and are not likely to be overturned in the near future.

CHAPTER 4

ORGANIZED STRUCTURES WITHIN HOSPITALS

Medical Staff Structures

To understand how peer review works, it is important to be familiar with medical staff structures. Physicians with privileges at a hospital are considered members of the medical staff. The medical staff is a formal structure made up of physician departments divided by specialties, such as departments of medicine, surgery, anesthesiology, obstetrics, and pediatrics. Specific departments and their structures are determined by the size and scope of services offered at the hospital.

The authority over the specialty department and the medical staff is the medical executive committee (MEC).[1] The MEC is generally made up of the chairs of each department and a number of ad hoc (specially elected or appointed) physician members. It has formal responsibility for physician credentialing, peer review, policy setting, utilization of physician services, medical education, and quality-improvement activities.

Medical Staff Officers

A hospital's medical staff bylaws set forth the structure for its medical staff officers. Members of the medical staff have nominating and voting rights. The medical staff has an elected chief of staff, who serves a one- to two-year term. In addition, each formal department has a chief or chair, who also serves a one- to two-year term. Medical staffs have additional committees to oversee quality, credentialing, pharmacy services, laboratory reviews, medical records, continuing medical education, and physician well-being. The well-being committee deals with issues of behavior as well as personal substance abuse involving physicians.

Each individual medical staff department has closed physician committee meetings, meaning that the meetings are not open to the public, nor are they usually open to the hospital staff, other clinicians, or administrators. In each of these committees, medical staff members are assigned to review patient cases, screening for potential adverse events that may be related to the physician's management of the patient.

In these reviews, a patient's medical record, perhaps an incident report or patient complaint, and the applicable diagnostic tests comprise the information that the doctors evaluate. The physician involved in the patient's care may be a member of the committee, but a physician does not review his or her own cases. Physician peer reviewers gather facts and draw conclusions based on their clinical expertise and the evidence at hand.

In many cases the committee will communicate with the doctor involved in the case, or, if the doctor is not present, they may ask him or her to appear at a future meeting to give further input. The committee then assigns a rating to determine if the case met the standard of care. Medical staffs use various scoring methods for this, such as number, letter, or category scales. The concept can be best described as a "report card" methodology.

The medical staff operates under a set of bylaws, in addition to a set of preestablished rules and regulations, to reach a formal edict. Ultimate accountability for the functions of the medical staff falls to the hospital's governing board, which holds the medical staff responsible for adhering to its own medical staff bylaws, rules, and regulations. However, most hospital boards delegate the responsibility for physician functions, including peer review, to the MEC. Board members usually do not see, nor do they participate in, the peer-review discussions or actions. Boards may receive general trend reports on peer-review activities; some state regulations actually mandate that boards receive these reports. The hospital board will be involved with and must ratify medical staff decisions if the peer-review process leads to permanent removal of a physician's clinical privileges.

Credentialing

Hospital boards, medical staff leaders, and hospital executives are responsible for ensuring that competent and proficient physicians practice at their hospital. It is easier to screen a physician before he or she joins the medical staff than it is to remove clinical privileges after a physician joins. The process that assures physicians are competent to join a hospital's medical staff is called credentialing. Credentialing is an extensive process during which the qualifications of a licensed physician are assessed and confirmed. Physicians must provide a number of verification items, including but not limited to physician education, license status, type of skill set, training, certified references, and board certification.

The credentialing process begins when a physician files an application for privileges at a particular hospital. The hospital runs queries on the physician from the NPDB to confirm that a physician is in good standing. These queries verify the information the physician supplied on his or her application as well as his or her board certification status, malpractice litigation history, and active federal Drug Enforcement Administration (DEA) registration, allowing physicians to dispense controlled substances such as narcotics.

Board Certification

Board certification is a rigorous process that requires additional education and training in the applied specialty as well as an intensive oral and written examination in that selected area of expertise. In addition, continuing education is required to maintain board certification, which is usually renewable every six years. Each specialty has specific standards for certification. Twenty-four physician specialties provide board certification (see table of board certification specialties).

After receipt of information and once the source verification is completed, the physician is notified of one of the following:

1. The physician is granted clinical privileges or appointed to the medical staff.
2. The physician is required to submit further information.
3. The physician is disqualified because credentialing requirements were not met.

Tips

A number of hospitals post their bylaws, rules, and regulations on the Internet. Initiate an Internet search on medical staff bylaws and you

Table 4.1
Board Certification Specialties

Board Certification
Allergy and immunology
Anesthesiology
Colon and rectal surgery
Dermatology
Emergency medicine
Family practice
Internal medicine
Medical genetics
Neurological surgery
Nuclear medicine
Obstetrics and gynecology
Orthopaedic surgery
Otolaryngology
Pathology
Pediatrics
Physical medicine and rehabilitation
Plastic surgery
Preventative medicine
Psychiatry and neurology
Radiology
Surgery
Thoracic surgery
Urology

Source: Created from American Board of Medical
Specialties (2004).

can read the details behind many bylaws. A few examples are listed here:
http://mga.dhs.state.br.us/QMWeb/MedDirection.htm, http://www.
aapsonline. org/bylaws.htm.

Before selecting a new physician, inquire whether he or she is board
certified.

Board certification is an extensive process for physicians. Consider
using board-certified physicians. Keep in mind that although board
certification helps to qualify a physician's training and expertise, it
does not guarantee competence. Use board certification in conjunction
with the physician's experience and training and recommendations
from other physicians and health care providers.

A hospital credentials a physician for a two-year period. During this span an active staff physician must complete some or all of the following requirements to remain credentialed:

- A predesignated number of patient admissions or procedures (depending on the physician's specialty).
- Attendance at a set number of medical staff and peer review meetings delineated in the medical staff bylaws.
- Achievement and maintenance of good standing for completion of patient medical records. When a patient is discharged from the hospital, the medical record must include a dictated physician history and physical, a discharge summary of clinical care provided to the hospitalized patient, and a report of each procedure or surgery, all within a specified time. Before a patient medical record is considered complete, the doctor must dictate and sign all of these patient dictations. Full billing cannot occur until these dictations are completed and signed. Physicians can be suspended for not completing records on time, although this suspension is administrative rather than clinical; the physician may lose admitting privileges until his or her patient dictation reports are current.

Continuing Medical Education for Doctors

Physicians must complete continuing medical education credits, known as CMEs. Requirements for continuing medical education credits vary by state, ranging from 12 to 50 hours per licensing period for each physician. Some states, such as Texas and Florida, require select types of course studies. Texas requires one of the 24 required CME hours to be in the study of bioethics; Florida requires courses in HIV and domestic violence.

Tip

To view the continuing medical education requirements for each state, log on to www.ama-assn.org/ama/upload/mm/40/table14.pdf.

Physician Profiles

The hospital's quality department monitors the physician during the two years by the use of a physician profile consisting of process, outcome, and financial indicators. In addition to these quality indicators, error data, often in the form of incident reports, are integrated into the physician profile. A sample hospital physician profile is included at the end of this chapter.

Content of the profiles varies, but standard information includes volume rates, such as how many open-heart procedures a cardiac surgeon performed; complication rates, such as unplanned returns to the operating room; bleeding rates; and infections. Doctors are compared to their peers in the profile.

Recredentialing

Peers evaluate the physician's recredentialing file before the expiration of his or her privileges. If clinical problems develop within the two-year time frame, those issues are picked up through clinical data as well as verbal and written complaints. The issues are dealt with accordingly.

On the approval of the clinical specialty committee, the physician file is forwarded to the credentialing committee, and if approved, the file goes to the MEC. Accrediting organizations, as well as state medical boards, strictly enforce the two-year credentialing period.

Challenges of Removing a Physician's Privileges

How does a medical staff handle incompetent or impaired physicians, especially since the doctors police their own work? It is not easy. Once a physician is granted privileges, or is credentialed, at a hospital, it is a complicated and extensive process to remove those clinical privileges. The formal structure of medical staff bylaws and state medical board regulations afford physicians protective rights.

THE CASE OF DR. D

Seems Simple

Dr. D, age 61, was an obstetrician who practiced in a local Texas community. He had clinical privileges at two area hospitals, although most of his practice had been focused at one hospital. His partner had recently retired, and he began to see more patients. He decided to increase his practice at the second hospital.

One night in late January, a patient of Dr. D's was having a difficult labor. The nurses tried to reach Dr. D and became frustrated as they called him several times with no response. After several hours, he finally returned their calls and came to the hospital.

The baby to be delivered was larger than expected. After a high forceps delivery, a 10-pound, eight-ounce baby girl was born. The baby was transferred to the high-risk nursery. Several hours after the delivery, the baby became lethargic and sleepy. The nurses checked the blood sugar and it was 39. A normal range is between 70 and 100, so an intravenous (IV) line with glucose was started, because the baby was too weak to take a bottle. The baby became active again. A blood sugar test was repeated and it was 89.

The nurses were concerned by the events that occurred, so they completed an incident report. The quality department received the report, and the director of quality remembered a similar event that had taken place with one of Dr. D's patients two months earlier. The director took her concerns about the two cases to the chief of obstetrics. The two ran some internal reports and found that several of Dr. D's patients had difficult deliveries with large infants, followed by newborn low blood sugar.

The chief of the department set up a meeting with Dr. D to review the findings. Dr. D explained that in his practice he treated some Hispanic mothers who traveled from Mexico and who had often received little or no early prenatal care. These moms were at high risk for developing diabetes during pregnancy, known as gestational diabetes mellitus (GDM). He had not screened these moms for this, since they had seen him only a few weeks before their delivery. He felt that undetected gestational diabetes and late prenatal care led to the larger babies and infant low blood sugar after birth. The chief accepted this explanation. However, he encouraged Dr. D to promptly return nurses' calls from the hospital. Dr. D assured the chief that he would always do this.

Several weeks later, Dr. D had another patient with a baby who developed low blood sugar soon after delivery. The nurses filed an incident report. The quality director once again spoke with the chief of obstetrics. The decision was made to do an informal review of Dr. D's cases. The data were prepared and the information was taken to the obstetrics peer review committee. In a closed session, the physicians confirmed that Dr. D was not screening all of his patients for gestational diabetes; hence, these complications were occurring.

The committee elected to invite Dr. D to the next peer review meeting, in May. The medical staff office contacted Dr. D, but he was leaving on a previously planned trip to Europe, so he was unable to attend until June.

During that interim, another patient of Dr. D's delivered a large baby born with shoulder dystocia (a weak shoulder, sometimes caused by an injury during birth) after a difficult delivery. The quality department added this case to Dr. D's file.

In June, Dr. D appeared before the obstetrics peer review committee. The committee discussed with him its findings and concerns. However, Dr. D brought along several of his office records that confirmed his patients came to him late in their pregnancies and were not screened for gestational diabetes. Dr. D also explained that his retired partner had employed a nurse who had arranged the diabetes screenings. Since his partner had retired, the nurse had also left, and Dr. D had not set up a new screening process. Dr. D promised that in the future he would be more diligent in screening for gestational diabetes and that he would manage infant deliveries more appropriately. The committee accepted this.

Over the next three months, Dr. D had two more cases of newborn low blood sugar, one in which it was difficult to revive the baby. These cases were reported through incident reports filed by the nurses and added to Dr. D's file.

The obstetrics committee met in September and decided to perform a special chart review on all of Dr. D's deliveries. Two obstetricians, Dr. B and Dr. F, were assigned to review Dr. D's cases over the next three months. The special chart review proceeded, and a letter explaining the review was sent to Dr. D.

Following this, there was another case of shoulder dystocia, this time with nerve damage to the baby's hand. During the special review of Dr. D's cases Dr. B and Dr. F discovered from other hospital records that two of Dr. D's previous patients had come to Dr. D early in their pregnancies and could have been screened for gestational diabetes.

The committee asked Dr. D to appear again to explain the discrepancies; however, it was now December and the committee was not meeting again until after the first of the year.

Dr. D appeared at the January committee meeting and did not have a reasonable explanation for the two patient discrepancies, other than "the hospital records must be wrong." The committee decided to continue the special case review.

In February, another baby was delivered by Dr. D using forceps. Although the baby boy was not large, he had several deep lacerations on his head and developed temporary breathing problems after delivery. The nurses filed yet another incident report.

In March, the obstetrics committee met and reviewed all the patient records. The peers were clearly concerned about Dr. D's competency. The obstetrics committee recommended to the chief of staff that Dr. D appear before the MEC. According to the medical staff bylaws, Dr. D was entitled to have an attorney and one other representative present.

Dr. D appeared before the MEC with his attorney and a highly respected obstetrician from the community who had previously worked with Dr. D. The respected physician gave Dr. D a glowing review alluding to the expert care he provided for his patients.

The members of the MEC listened to the witness and the members found they had mixed feelings about Dr. D's performance. They felt bad for Dr. D because he was getting on in years. The committee recommended that the obstetrics committee continue to monitor him, but they did not formally sanction the special chart review, which later they discovered was a requirement set forth in one of their medical staff policies.

In May, Dr. D performed an extremely difficult delivery, and the baby was born dead. The nurses were outraged and brought their concerns directly to the chief of staff. He and the chief of the obstetrics committee called an emergency session of the MEC. The committee reviewed the infant death and recommended a summary suspension, or revocation of clinical privileges for Dr. D.

According to the medical staff bylaws, the hospital needed to notify Dr. D in writing within 24 hours of the summary suspension, outlining the reasons for the suspension. The MEC also had to decide how long to suspend Dr. D's privileges, knowing that if the suspension was longer than 30 days, it must report it to the National Practitioner Data Bank.

The medical staff bylaws stated that before the length of the summary suspension was determined, Dr. D was entitled to a hearing within one week of the time he received the notification of the suspension.

The hospital set up a hearing for Dr. D with an officer from the State Medical Board assigned to oversee the proceedings. All of this was quickly arranged.

The chief of staff and the medical staff attorney appointed five members of the medical staff who had not been involved with the patient record reviews or any meetings regarding Dr. D's cases. The panel was selected much like a jury is chosen, assuring impartiality.

The hearing began and the medical staff attorney presented the history, case records, and findings to the hearing panel. The medical staff attorney outlined all the events that led up to the summary suspension.

In response, Dr. D's attorney presented his defense as follows:

1. *The summary suspension was imposed on Dr. D not to improve patient-care quality, but rather to sanction the following financial limitations on his practice:*

   a. *Dr. B and Dr. F, the physicians who performed the special record review, are two of Dr. D's greatest competitors for patients in this part of the community.*

   b. *Two years ago, Dr. D superseded the chief of obstetrics in winning one of the largest insurance contracts in the local community, and the chief of obstetrics is looking for retaliation against Dr. D. The chief has done the review not to improve quality, but to seek revenge.*

   c. *The concentrated review done on Dr. D failed to use outside physician reviewers, either from another neutral hospital or from the State Medical Board. Biased parties did the review.*

2. *The MEC had not initially sanctioned the special record review. (Dr. D's attorney reviewed the medical staff bylaws and found a policy that stated that any special review had to be formally approved through voting by the MEC. This had not been done.) He stated again, "The obstetrics committee was targeting Dr. D for competitive financial reasons and their motive was not to improve quality." They did this without oversight from the MEC.*

3. *The mother of the baby who died had an extensive history of cocaine use, and the baby's death was related to the mother's drug abuse, not medical mismanagement. Dr. D's attorney presented a toxicology report that showed trace elements of cocaine in the mother's bloodstream at the time of delivery.*

4. Dr. D's attorney brought forth the highly respected community obstetrician, who again testified on Dr. D's stellar patient care.

The medical staff panel deliberated for 30 minutes and overturned the summary suspension. The hearing officer ratified the decision. One week later, Dr. D stated he was retiring from practice at that hospital and resigned his clinical privileges.

Although he continued to practice at the other hospital, none of the information on Dr. D was reported to the State Medical Board or to the NPDB. There was no requirement that the hospital report its findings to those organizations or to the other community hospital. No law required outside reporting of Dr. D's actions, and peer-review laws protected the proceedings and records concerning Dr. D.

Because of the alleged financial motivation of Dr. D's peers, the medical staff was concerned about taking any further action that might bring a lawsuit against them by Dr. D for "financially punishing" him.

Just as the U.S. judicial system affords many rights that can affect outcomes of legal proceedings, physicians are afforded rights, and they can use several aspects of these rights to defend their clinical privileges. Hence, stating that a doctor is incompetent can be difficult to prove even with valid evidence.

Hiring Doctors

Physicians can be hired by hospitals as medical directors. Some states set up parameters to regulate how hiring is defined. The medical directors may be limited to the number of hours and scope of service they perform so as not to create conflicts of interest. The medical directors are often contracted; sometimes report to the hospital's chief executive officer; and have a clear scope of responsibility such as medical director of critical care, pediatrics, or utilization review. Medical directors also have clinical privileges, which are entirely independent of their contracted work. A medical director can leave or be terminated according to his or her contract, but this does not automate removal of clinical privileges from the medical staff.[2]

Medical directors are generally paid market value for their services. Department chairs often receive little or no monetary compensation for their one- to two-year terms. Medical chiefs of staff receive either very small stipends or no compensation for their terms. Being the chief of staff can be a grueling experience. For those physicians their terms require them to divert their focus away from patient care. They risk decreasing their patient base during their terms and then having to rebuild it again afterward. For the most part, serving as the chief of staff is a financial risk for physicians, and it is truly voluntary in many regards.

Tip

If you have a complaint against your doctor about care you receive while in the hospital, first speak with your doctor. If the matter is not settled, then address your concern to the chief of the department or the chief of staff. The medical staff will review the case, but you will not have access to information about any actions taken against the doctor.

Figure 4.1
Joe Cardiac Surgeon Recredentialing File, 2002–2004

Active Staff, Years on staff: 8
License number: AZ. 123456
Thoracic Surgeon   Board Certified: No

Admissions/ Procedures	Number of cases/ Totals	Patient's average days in hospital	Bleeding complications	Returns to the operating room	Surgical site Infections	To the hospital	Death rate	Operating room death
Coronary artery bypass (CABG) surgeries	100	8	20%	15%	4%	6%	5%	1%
Heart valve	30	9					10%	0
CABG/valve	21	11	25%	10%	10%		10%	5%
Other procedures	6	4					0	0
Incident reports filed on cases	27		20					
Blood product use	39							
Adverse drug events	18							
Cases outside the standard of clinical care	5		3	1	1			
Violation of physician behavior	7							
Recommend reappointment	Cardiac committee	Surgery committee	Credentialing committee	Quality committee	Medical executive committee			Reappointed
	Y	Y	Y	N	Y			Y 10/04

Average Physician Peer Comparison Recredentialing File 2002-2004

Admissions/ Procedures	Number of cases/ Totals	Average days in hospital	Bleeding complications	Returns to operating room	Surgical site Infections	Readmits to the hospital	Death rate	Operating room death
Coronary artery bypass surgeries	82	6	4%	5%	1%	1%	2%	0
Heart valve	19	7					5%	0
CABG/valve	15	8	8%	6%	2%		4%	1%
Other procedures	12	3					0	0
Average Incident reports filed on peers	4							
Blood-use	6							
Adverse drug events	3							
Cases outside the standard of clinical care	1							
Violation of physician behavior standard	1							

CHAPTER 5

WHO IS WATCHING THE HOSPITALS?

Joint Commission on Accreditation of Healthcare Organizations

The Joint Commission on Accreditation of Healthcare Organizations (JCAHO) is an organization that accredits 95 percent of U.S. hospitals. Its purpose is to hold accredited hospitals accountable for safety and quality through a survey process. The JCAHO defines its mission as to "continuously improve the safety and quality of care provided to the public through the provision of health care accreditation and related services that support performance improvement in health care organizations."[1]

Hospitals accredited by the JCAHO undergo an intense on-site scheduled survey, carried out by a team of JCAHO surveyors, every three years. The hospital is held accountable for meeting a comprehensive set of standards that cover safety, quality, medical staff, leadership, governance, employees, patient care, environment, infection control, and information technology. In recent years, the JCAHO modified its standards to incorporate more patient safety standards after the release of the Institute of Medicine's 1999 report "To Err Is Human" (see chapter 1).

The JCAHO does not consider itself a regulatory agency, even though accredited hospitals are accountable for their actions, or lack of actions, under the standards it sets forth. The standards on safety are integrated throughout the JCAHO standard book and include the following sections: the leaders' role in safety, patient disclosure, data collection, root cause analysis, sentinel events, failure mode analysis, and environmental and equipment safety.

In 2004, the JCAHO is revamping its hospital survey process to move toward unannounced surveys. In discussing the new survey process, Dennis S. O'Leary, M.D., president of the JCAHO, states, "This creates the expectation that each accredited organization be in compliance with 100 percent of the Joint Commission's standards 100 percent of the time." The hospitals will not always have the year lead time to get into compliance with the standards, as they do presently.[2]

Accreditation is critical to hospitals, as Medicare and Medicaid funding often can be linked to accreditation standings. According to the JCAHO, a hospital may receive any of the following standings as a result of the hospital survey:

- Accreditation with Full Standards Compliance
- Accreditation with Requirements for Improvement
- Provisional Accreditation
- Conditional Accreditation
- Preliminary Denial of Accreditation
- Accreditation Denied
- Accreditation Watch[3]

Failure to be accredited will open the hospital up to scrutiny by the State Department of Health and the State Medical Board and make possible financial investigations, and often this will bring unwanted local media attention. Denial of accreditation may result in the closure of a hospital. However, it is not a frequent occurrence.[4] The JCAHO defines the following as accreditation denial:

- A decision that results when a health care organization has been denied accreditation.
- A health care organization fails to demonstrate compliance with applicable JCAHO standards in multiple performance areas.
- A health care organization is persistently unable or unwilling to demonstrate satisfactory compliance with one or more JCAHO standards.
- A health care organization fails to comply with one or more specified accreditation policy requirements, though it is believed to be capable of achieving acceptable compliance within a stipulated time period.

Problem areas delineated in conditional accreditation must be rapidly corrected, or accreditation denial will result. This accreditation decision becomes effective only when all available appeal procedures have been exhausted.

The highest accreditation score is the following:

Accreditation with Full Standards Compliance (formerly Accreditation without Type I Recommendations). This is an accreditation decision awarded to a health care organization that demonstrates satisfactory compliance with applicable JCAHO standards in all performance areas.

The next and most common accreditation status is the following:

Accreditation with Type I Recommendation(s). A Type I recommendation requires the health care organization to resolve insufficient or unsatisfactory standards compliance in a specific performance area through a written progress report or during an unscheduled survey.

Survey scores range up to 100 percent. Scores in the 70th percentile indicate problems with survey results; hospitals strive for scores in the 90s. The majority of hospitals receive some Type I recommendations. A Type I recommendation may represent a problem as minor as staff not checking logs frequently enough or, at the other end of the spectrum, as serious as a violation of patient rights.

Accreditation is a comprehensive process. Nevertheless, even with this extensive survey process, areas can be missed. The survey team is at the hospital for only three to five days depending on the hospital's size. Not all documents are reviewed, and hospitals know what to highlight for the JCAHO surveyors.

Tip

The JCAHO provides brochures in both English and Spanish for the public on its hospital-accreditation process. See the organization's Web site, www. jcaho.org.

Sentinel Events and Root Cause Analysis

In 1998, the JCAHO defined the term *sentinel event* as a significant event experienced in a hospital that results in serious harm or death to a patient. Its formal definition is as follows: "A sentinel event is an unexpected occurrence involving death or serious physical or psychological injury, or the risk thereof. Serious injury specifically includes loss of limb or function. The phrase 'or the risk thereof' includes any process variation for which a recurrence would carry a significant chance of a serious adverse outcome. *Such events are called 'sentinel' because they signal the need for immediate investigation and response.*"[5]

The JCAHO requires that hospitals address sentinel events, and it allows hospitals to choose one of four alternatives for reporting them. Under the alternatives, hospitals are required to perform a root cause analysis. This is a thorough investigation of the circumstances that led to the adverse event, and it provides the best way to uncover latent conditions and other process errors. Root cause analysis is a technique used in aviation, including space travel, engineering, and the nuclear industry, to study accidents. This form of analysis has helped to bring about improvements in quality and patient safety, but trend data from root cause analyses needs to be used on a larger scale and in coordination with analyses from other hospitals. More about this will be discussed in chapter 11.

MR. L

A Direct Injection

In Louisiana, Mr. L, a 71-year-old patient, was having trouble with swelling; he was retaining too much body fluid, and the fluid was affecting his breathing. The doctor ordered an IV drug called Lasix, which causes the body to eliminate extra fluid, to help Mr. L breathe more easily. The nurse took the medication to the patient's room and injected the medicine into the IV port. Within a minute of the injection, Mr. L went into cardiac arrest. The staff called a code and attempted to resuscitate him, but six hours later he died. The nurse had mixed up the vials and had given Mr. L a lethal injection of potassium chloride.[6]

Root Causes

Numerous root cause analyses, performed over time and at different hospitals, have led to a major change in the storage and preparation of potassium chloride in an attempt to avoid this mistake. The results of the various root cause analyses showed that the foremost reason for this error was the similarity of potassium chloride vials to those containing Lasix. The death of Mr. L occurred in 1996. Unfortunately, the requirement to remove concentrated potassium from patient care areas, so as to avoid mix-ups, was not imposed on hospitals until January 2003. At the time of Mr. L's death, the

Institute of Safe Medication Practices had reports of at least 12 other deaths from accidental overdoses of potassium.[7] Why did it take seven years to mandate a stop to the practice of storing concentrated potassium in patient care areas where it was easily accessible and easy to mix up with Lasix, a commonly used drug for fluid elimination?

Speaking Up

Dr. Michael Leonard, an anesthesiologist and chief of surgery at a Colorado hospital, was operating on a patient when he reached into a drawer for medicine. Inside were two vials, side by side. Both had yellow labels. Both had yellow caps. One was a paralyzing agent, which Dr. Leonard had correctly administered to keep the patient still during the operation. The other was the reversal agent, which he needed next. "I grabbed the wrong one," Dr. Leonard recalled. "I used the wrong drug."

It would have been easy for the doctor to keep quiet; the drug wore off and the patient was not harmed. Instead, he talked—to the surgeon and scrub nurses, the patient's wife, and the hospital pharmacist, who has since relabeled the paralyzing agents with red stickers and put them in a separate drawer. He also talked to his five partners, whose reaction unnerved him.

"Four of the five of them said, 'You know, I've done the same thing,' Dr. Leonard said. "One of them said, 'I did the same thing last week.' And I'm thinking, I've been chief of this department for five years. Now I'm chief of surgery. And nobody has ever said to me, 'We have this problem.' A lot of it comes back to this culture of silence.[8]

By speaking up, Dr. Leonard was able to identify a problem and avert future such episodes. Both Dr. Leonard's case and the case in Louisiana warrant thorough root cause analysis to determine all the latent conditions in the processes that led up to active errors. An effective root cause analysis guides a hospital to make immediate changes in processes causing adverse events.

Tip

To learn more about root cause analysis see the JCAHO publication *Root Cause Analysis in Health Care.* Oak Terrace. See www.jcrinc.com.

Reporting Sentinel Events

The mandatory sharing of root cause analyses among hospitals can only help to enhance patient safety. Nevertheless, the reporting of

Figure 5.1
Root Cause Analysis

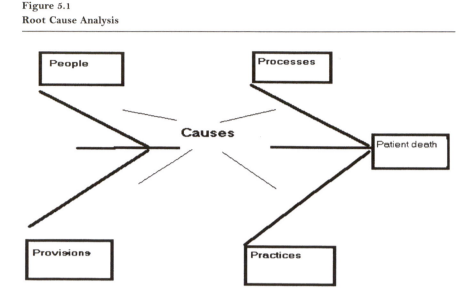

sentinel events and the sharing of root cause analyses is still a voluntary practice by hospitals. As mentioned earlier, as of 2000 accredited hospitals are now required to preselect one of the four alternatives for voluntarily reporting sentinel events and notify the JCAHO of their selection.

MRS. GREENWOOD

A Sentinel Event: Giving a Medication the Wrong Way

In a Georgia hospital, Mrs. Greenwood, age 62, was being treated for heart problems. She also had an order written for a medicine to calm her stomach. This medicine was a milky mixture that Mrs. Greenwood's nurse had never given before. When the medicine arrived on the floor, the charge nurse handed the medicine to the nurse caring for Mrs. Greenwood. The nurse took the medicine without looking at the doctor's order. He assumed that the medicine was to be given intravenously. The nurse withdrew the medicine with a syringe from the bottle, took it to Mrs. Greenwood's bedside, and injected it into Mrs. Greenwood's IV line. Within a minute of the injection, Mrs. Greenwood grabbed her chest and said, "I can't breathe." She collapsed into cardiac arrest, in front of her son. The hospital code team tried to resuscitate Mrs. Greenwood but was unsuccessful. An autopsy later revealed that Mrs. Greenwood died of multiple small blood clots in her lungs caused by the medicine, which was not designed to be given intravenously. This was clearly a sentinel event.

The following are the choices that the JCAHO provides to hospitals for reporting sentinel events:[9]

JCAHO ALTERNATIVE 1

This alternative permits hospital representatives to schedule an appointment to personally bring the root cause analysis and other sentinel event–related documents to the JCAHO headquarters in Chicago for review by commission staff and then leave with all of these documents still in the hospital's possession.

In the case of the event involving Mrs. Greenwood, representatives from the hospital would take the investigational documents, including the root cause analysis and action plan documents about Mrs. Greenwood's death, to the JCAHO headquarters in Chicago. The commission would see all the information surrounding the death. This investigation would most likely prompt an on-site survey.

JCAHO ALTERNATIVE 2

Alternative 2 permits the organization to request an on-site review of the root cause analysis and other sentinel event–related documents by a JCAHO surveyor.

With alternative 2, the Georgia hospital would invite the JCAHO surveyors to come to the hospital to review all the investigational documents. The JCAHO would see the details of the mistake through the root cause analysis. This investigation would most likely prompt attention from the state for reporting adverse events resulting in harm or death and may lead to a citation and fine from the state for the hospital.

JCAHO ALTERNATIVE 3

Alternative 3 permits the organization to request an on-site visit by a JCAHO surveyor who will conduct interviews and review relevant documentation to obtain information about the process and findings of the root cause analysis and resulting action plan without actually reviewing the root cause analysis documents.

Under this alternative, the Georgia hospital would invite the JCAHO surveyors to come to the hospital. The survey team would look at the hospital's procedure for handling a sentinel event review, and it has an option to interview staff. Although surveyors do not look directly at the root cause analysis document, it is very likely they will discover the details surrounding Mrs. Greenwood's death through the interview process.

JCAHO ALTERNATIVE 4

Alternative 4 permits the hospital to request an on-site review of its process for responding to a sentinel event and relevant policies and procedures preceding and following the organization's review of the specific event.

In Mrs. Greenwood's case, the JCAHO would not review the actual death as long as it is satisfied that the hospital sentinel event process is sufficient to implement an action plan to make improvements.

Alternative 4 is the least restrictive selection (they review the least information), followed in increasing order of stringency by alternatives 3, 2, and 1, respectively. Because reporting is voluntary, the hospital is not obligated to invite JCAHO surveyors under any of the alternatives. In 2000, many of the hospitals in the United States selected the least restrictive alternatives for reporting sentinel events.

During the hospital's regularly scheduled accreditation survey, the surveyors will look at the hospital's process and policies for dealing with sentinel events, but the JCAHO may never know about injuries and deaths that may have occurred during the previous three years. In the event the JCAHO finds a significant event and defines it as a "reviewable" sentinel event, then the surveyors will take action to investigate both the process and the sentinel event.

Tip

The JCAHO maintains a Web site that the public can use to report concerns about hospitals: http://www.jcaho.org.

Sentinel Event Trends

The JCAHO receives only a small number of reports on injuries and deaths because the process is voluntary. The data that the commission collects is posted on its Web site. The JCAHO also creates sentinel event alerts, which notify hospitals about common types of sentinel events. Hospitals are then obligated to educate their staffs in methods of preventing the particular type of event discussed in the alert. The first sentinel event alert was published in February 1998. Topics of these alerts have included wrong site surgery, patient suicide, and infant abduction.

Table 5.1
Sentinel Events, January 1995 to June 2004

Total number of sentinel events January 1995 - June 2004	Total 2552

Type of Events	Number
Patient suicide	382
Surgical complication	330
Wrong site surgery	310
Medication error	291
Delay in treatment	172
Patient fall	114
Restraints, patient death/injury	113
Assault	89
Transfusion error	73
Infant death/loss of function	71
Breathing equipment death/injury	39
Anesthesia-related event	38
Infection-related event	38
Medical equipment-related event	33
Maternal death	31
Other	428
Total	**2552**

Sentinel event outcomes	
Patient death	2000
Loss of function	268
Other	399
Total patients impacted	2667
* Note: more than one patient can be impacted by each sentinel event	

	Non self reported	Self reported
Self reported vs. non-self reported	864	1688

Sources of sentinel event identification	Number	Percentage
Self reported	1688	66%
Complaints	270	11%
Media	257	10%
Found during JCAHO survey	190	7%
Other regulatory agencies' reports	147	6%

Source: Joint Commission on Accreditation of Health Care Organizations (2004).

In comparison to the IOM report, stating that between 44,000 and 98,000 people die annually as a result of medical errors, injuries and deaths seem to be "voluntarily" unreported to the JCAHO and other regulatory agencies. Hence, this data cannot be compared to the IOM report. Sadly, this underreporting limits the full scope of error prevention that could otherwise occur from comprehensive data.

Moving Forward

In these chapters I have outlined multiple reasons that the public does not see what lies beneath the surface of the medical error iceberg. The HCQIA legislation was originally designed to improve quality, but it has not met its objective. The Institute of Medicine, along with studies carried out by numerous other researchers, confirms we are experiencing a crisis of patient harm. People in medicine do not intend to inflict harm; on the contrary, most of them go into health care to help others. Nevertheless, physicians and health care professionals are working in systems that are outdated; fragmented; and, frankly, just plain dangerous. Moving beyond the silence, in a reasonable fashion that will promote patient safety and diminish harm, is the first step in reducing medical errors. The informed consumer can assist in preventing some medical injuries and mishaps and, most importantly, can help to point out latent conditions, dangers, and potential broken barriers that may lead to patient harm.

CHAPTER 6

MAKING SAFER HEALTH CARE CHOICES: WHAT THE NUMBERS MEAN

MR. D

Do Health Care Report Cards Tell the Whole Story?

After undergoing a cardiac catheterization, Mr. D was told by his cardiologist that he had two partially blocked coronary arteries and that he needed open-heart bypass surgery. The cardiologist said that it was not an emergency, but Mr. D should have the surgery within the next few weeks.

Mr. D, a businessman in Chicago, belonged to a health plan that allowed him to select among six cardiac surgeons. To help in his decision, he logged onto a Web site that provided public data on surgeons. After evaluating the doctors' profiles, Mr. D narrowed his selection to three cardiac surgeons. Each one was rated on a scale of one to five (five being the best rating) in categories including type of cardiac surgeries performed, cardiac procedures including angioplasty, and quality of care. Each of the three had at least one score of five. Mr. D decided to interview the three doctors to select the best one.

At the first physician's office, Mr. D found the surgeon extremely rushed and rather rude. He crossed that doctor off his list.

When Mr. D tried to schedule an interview with the second doctor, the staff initially hesitated to make an appointment for just an interview. "Honey, the doctor is far too busy," he was told. Mr. D explained why it was important for him to interview the doctor, and the staff finally made the appointment.

When Mr. D arrived at the office he waited almost two hours for his appointment without any explanation of the delay. Although the doctor seemed pleasant enough, the surgeon's staff treated Mr. D as if he was in the way. Mr. D decided against this doctor because of the rudeness of the office staff.

Then Mr. D met with the third surgeon. The staff was helpful and the surgeon was pleasant and kind. Mr. D selected this doctor and was scheduled for the procedure on the following Monday.

The initial surgery seemed to go well, but three hours after Mr. D was put into the surgical intensive care unit, his blood pressure fell rapidly. The surgeon was paged, and Mr. D was taken back to surgery for abnormal bleeding. The incision was reopened and the bleeding was controlled. Mr. D returned to the intensive care unit.

Again, Mr. D's blood pressure dropped, and he was rushed back to surgery. The surgeon had to reopen the chest incision to stop the bleeding. Mr. D was given two transfusions of red blood cells and required several additional medications. All of this resulted in several extra days in the intensive care unit.

What happened? Mr. D seemed to have done his homework.

What Mr. D did not know about his surgeon was that he had been monitored through peer review for an abnormally high rate of patients returning to the operating room for bleeding complications. The hospital surgery peer review committee had reviewed the surgeon for the last two years after one of his surgical patients died from bleeding complications.

The peer review consisted of a detailed retrospective patient chart review. It appeared from the review that the surgeon's patients were older and sicker than his colleagues' patients, and this was the reason for the returns to the operating room. The surgeon was reprimanded by his peers and told to be more careful and not to operate on such "old, sick" patients.

The surgeon was never observed for his technique in surgery, which ultimately was the real reason for the high bleeding rates. This was later determined by peer review and direct observation by another cardiac surgeon. Because no formal action was taken against the surgeon, the hospital was not required to report the outcomes of peer review. The bleeding complications were not listed on the public database that Mr. D reviewed.

Tip

When evaluating data on a Web site, review publicly reported data carefully. Draw on other resources as well concerning the physician's expertise, experience, board certification, and use of reliable references. Be aware that public data give limited evaluation of a physician's performance and are vulnerable to misinterpretation.

Data Collection by Hospitals

Hospitals in the United States collect extraordinary volumes of data, including peer review indicators, studies on patient diseases, death rates by type of illness, adverse drug reaction rates, medication use, hospital-associated infection rates, surgical site infection rates, blood utilization data, anesthesia complications, surgical complications, patient fall rates, length of time (by days) patients stay in the hospital, patients readmitted to the hospital for complications, cesarean section rates, infant mortality, misread X-ray rates, patient delays, restraint use, patient satisfaction rates, financial utilization data, and numerous other rates and outcomes.

Data collected are categorized by different terms, including outcome, process, quality, clinical, and financial. An example of outcome data would be death rates for heart attack patients in the hospital. An example of process data would be how many heart attack patients were given aspirin while in the hospital (which is a recommended national best practice). Outcome and process data fall into a larger category called clinical data. Quality data include both clinical and financial data.

Quality Data, One Example

Hospitals continually aim to improve care for their patients through both quality and cost perspectives. Acute myocardial infarction, or heart attack, is one of the leading illnesses treated in U.S. hospitals.[1] The American Heart Association, in conjunction with the American College of Cardiology, established guidelines for care that recommend best-practice treatments for patients with heart attacks. Consequently, individual hospitals should and often do determine their compliance with the recommended best practice, and they collect and analyze data.

Table 6.1
Categories with Examples of Data That Hospitals Collect

Quality data			
Clinical data		**Financial data**	
Process data	**Outcome data**	**Process data**	**Outcome data**
Aspirin given to heart attack patients in the hospital	Death rates of heart attack patients within the hospital	Cost of nursing care	Did hospital meet annual budget?

Table 6.2
Hospital X: Aspirin Use in Heart Attack Patients within the Hospital Visit

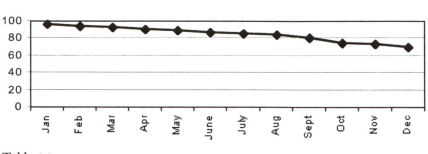

Percentage of Heart Attack Patients Given Aspirin

Table 6.3
Hospital X: Death Rate in Heart Attack Patients within the Hospital

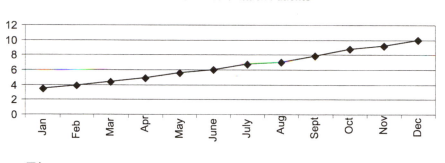

Death Rate in Heart Attack Patients

Tip

To view the American Heart Association's recommendations for the treatment of heart attack, log on to the AHA Web site at http://www. ahajournals.org.

In view of the American Heart Association's recommendation that most heart attack patients receive aspirin (aspirin has been proven to decrease death rates in heart attack patients), hospital X needs to analyze its downward trend of aspirin use. This rate, often referred to as an indicator, is not in itself sufficient data to explain the facts surrounding the treatment of heart attack patients. The hospital needs to collect more indicators, then evaluate and analyze them together to see if a correlation exists between the decreasing rate of aspirin use and the increasing death rate among hospital X's heart attack patients.

Many reasons may exist for these two trends: Perhaps the heart attack patients coming to the hospital in the last half of the year had chronic illnesses such as diabetes. Diabetes can predispose a heart attack patient to a higher mortality rate. Or perhaps those patients waited longer to come to the hospital after their symptoms started. Waiting to be treated when having a heart attack increases a patient's chances of dying. Conceivably, the average age of the patients in the second half of the year could have been much older compared to the patients who came in the first half of the year, and the mortality rate is higher in older adults. The only way to confirm the reasons for the trends is to collect additional indicators on these patients including chronic illnesses, average time patients waited to come to the hospital, and average age.

Reasons Hospital Data Are Not Reported to the Public

Given that hospitals collect huge volumes of data on diseases and physicians, why are these data not available to the public? Outside of physician peer-review protection, there are several reasons for this. The most compelling reason is the fear of misinterpretation of the data by the public. Using heart attack patients as an example, when an outside public or private organization creates a Web site to publish physician and hospital data, it usually has access to some but not all of the hospital indicators on heart attacks. Hence, the organization publishes what it does have, which may not represent the complete scope what actually transpired at the hospital. Consumers go to the Web site and see the reported heart attack death rate for hospital X, and they may draw a false conclusion about the hospital's care of heart attack patients. As discussed previously, the public may not have access to additional data on the patients who were treated. In the example of hospital X, patients who were treated later in the year did indeed have a higher prevalence of diabetes, waited longer to come to the hospital, and were older. Hence, the public may misinterpret the data: they see only hospital X's death rate, but they have no way of knowing the mitigating factors.

Tips

When looking at rates, always look at the numerator (the number of people being evaluated) and the denominator (the total number in the group). Rates by themselves can be deceptive.

When reviewing public data, always read the definitions thoroughly and determine how the data was obtained and analyzed.

If you or a family member is experiencing a heart attack, ask about the medications given immediately at the hospital. Ask specifically about aspirin, ACE inhibitors, and beta-blockers, which are recommended for most patients having a heart attack.

Note: Some patients may not be able to take all of these medications because of contraindications; it will be the physicians' decision. If one of the drugs is excluded, however, be sure to ask why. Do not assume that every heart attack patient is automatically going to receive all indicated medications.

Medicare and Medicaid Data

Currently, one of the core sources for publicly reported data consists of billing data. Medicare, now called the Center for Medicare and Medicaid, or CMS, collects and publishes data called Medicare Provider Analysis and Review (MEDPAR).

Tip

To learn more about MEDPAR data, log on to http://cms.hhs.gov/.

Effective October 1, 1983, Medicare implemented a prospective payment system (PPS) for reimbursing hospitals. This system replaced the existing retrospective cost reimbursement system whereby interim rates were paid on each bill. Most hospitals are now paid a fixed amount, determined in advance, for the costs of each case according to one of approximately 500 diagnosis-related groups (DRGs) such as colon surgery, heart attack, and hip replacement. Each patient discharge is assigned to a DRG based on diagnosis, surgery, patient age, discharge destination, and sex. Each DRG has a weight established for it based primarily on Medicare billing and cost data.

There are significant limitations to this available data. First, and most importantly, the available public data are designed for financial billing of medical care, not to evaluate sound clinical care. The information does not paint an accurate picture as to whether care was good or bad. Hence, the data can be misleading both in positive ways (e.g., overstating results) and in negative ways (e.g., missing valuable clinical components).

Another drawback of publicly reported data is that much of the data are old, generally more than two to three years. Hospitals may have made significant quality improvements in a three-year time frame, and the old data may not reflect the improvements.

Last, public sources of data usually do not cover all patients treated. Private insurance and HMO patients are often not included in publicly reported statistics, although some private insurance groups are launching initiatives to publicly report data.

Move to Publish Data on Patient Safety

The Leapfrog Group

There is a critical need for the medical industry to organize and validate health care data so consumers can draw accurate conclusions and make safer health choices. One of the leaders in the area of publicly reporting hospital data is the Leapfrog Group.

> The Leapfrog Group was created to help save lives and reduce preventable medical mistakes by mobilizing employer purchasing power to initiate breakthrough improvements in the safety of health care and by giving consumers information to make more informed hospital choices.[2]

Tip

To learn more about the Leapfrog Group log on to http://www.leapfroggroup.org/about.htm.

The Leapfrog Group was formed by the Business Roundtable, an association of the chief executive officers of leading U.S. corporations with a combined workforce of 10 million employees. The organization is committed to improving public policy. Large U.S. companies pay a significant portion of health insurance premiums. A goal of the Business Roundtable is to impact health care by promoting "incremental, market-based legislative reform of the U.S. health care system to maximize marketplace efficiency, quality, and coverage." The Leapfrog Group is intended to be one of the vehicles through which the Business Roundtable accomplishes this objective.

The Leapfrog Group's response toward the IOM's report "To Err Is Human" was to spotlight areas of quality by making "leaps" in safety through a Web-based survey of hospitals. The voluntary survey assesses three critical areas that have been shown through research literature to improve patient safety. These areas are as follows:

1. The use of electronic physician ordering systems, specifically the component called computerized physician order entry (CPOE).
2. The volume of select procedures that hospitals perform.
3. The use of intensive care physician programs within hospitals.[3]

From Handwriting to Computerized Physician Order Entry

The prescription shown in the first example resulted in the death of Ramon Vasquez, a Texas man. The prescription was written for

Example 6.1

Source: Institute for Safe Medication Practices, 16 July 1997 issue.

Example 6.2

Source: Institute of Safe Medication Practices, 3 October 2002 issue.

Example 6.3

Source: Institute of Safe Medication Practices, 3 October 2001. ismp.org.

the drug Pendil to help control Mr. Vasquez's blood pressure. The pharmacist misinterpreted the handwriting and dispensed the drug Isodil, a commonly used medication for treatment of chest pain. The problem was that the dose that was appropriate for the Pendil was 10 times the standard dose of Isodil. A day after taking the medication, Vasquez died of a heart attack.[4]

The second example was filled by a pharmacist as Anivert, an antihistamine that has been around for years. The medication actually intended was Axert, a drug for migraine headaches.

The third example was a mix-up in types of insulin. Instead of Lantus, which is a newer form of insulin, Lente, an older form of insulin, was dispensed. The patient took one dose of Lente with no adverse reaction.

Pharmacists and nurses in U.S. health care systems face the dilemma of interpreting handwritten orders on a regular basis. Computerized physician order entry (CPOE) is an electronic way to enter doctors' orders. An electronic ordering system significantly enhances the safety of physician orders. First and foremost, handwriting is eliminated. Once the order is entered, it is instantly transmitted to the pharmacist who will be filling the prescription and the nurses who will be administering the medications. This eliminates the paper trail and interpretation issues.

Additionally, CPOE systems provide alerts or "expert rules." An example of how an alert works may have prevented the error with Mrs. C (see chapter 3). When she was being prepared for her cardiac procedure, the initial orders would have been entered electronically with a CPOE. If an expert rule was in place, parameters that were preset in the computer would have cross-referenced the patient's age and checked whether Mrs. C had any chronic illnesses that might put her at risk for complications with the contrast dye. An alert would have appeared on the electronic computer order screen, in the form of a warning (or window) or reminder that stated, "Perform renal (kidney) panel blood work?" This would have prompted the doctor and other health care professionals to consider this option and might have guided the cardiologist to use less contrast dye or to dilute the contrast dye so Mrs. C could clear the substance through her kidneys. Most likely, the hospitalization for Mrs. C would have been avoided.

Tips

Ask your doctor to print all of your prescriptions. Check each and clarify the medication name, dosage, amount, and time.

Many states now require a consult with a pharmacist when a patient starts a new medicine. Always ask for this consult even if the pharmacy does not offer it.

Cost as a Hindrance

The cost of electronic medical record systems can range from several million dollars per hospital to upward of $100 million for large multihospital systems. Hospitals recognize the need for change, but they are attempting to balance huge financial requirements for CPOEs and electronic medical records (EMRs) with safety needs.

The Number of Procedures Performed by a Hospital

Medical studies confirm that physicians and hospitals that perform higher numbers of more extensive and high-risk surgeries, procedures, and treatments have better outcomes and are more expert than those that perform lower numbers of these procedures.

According to the Leapfrog Group, "Over 100 scientific studies have demonstrated a relationship between a hospital's annual number of certain high-risk treatments and procedures and patient outcomes. Patients who go to hospitals that frequently perform these high-risk treatments or procedures, or to hospitals that have demonstrated a good record for patient outcomes, have the best chance of surviving and successfully recovering."[5] Based on best-practice recommendations, Leapfrog set standards for recommended volumes of certain procedures, which are available on the organization's Web site.

Intensive Care Physicians

The third recommendation is the use of intensive care physicians. Technology, medicine, and treatments change rapidly, and it is extremely difficult for community physicians to stay current in all areas of practice. Intensive care physicians, also known as intensivists, treat people primarily within the hospital setting, and hence they can focus their practice and expertise in medicine on critically ill patients.

Intensivists are contracted by medical groups and hospitals to treat patients admitted to the hospital. Intensivist physician groups manage the care of patients from admission to discharge. These physicians are usually internal medicine physicians (not to be mistaken for interns) or pulmonologists, who specialize in the treatment of critical care including cardiac and lung diseases. The doctors are often board certified in their specialty.

According to a study from the American College of Physicians, "In the nine studies that met our selection criteria, relative reductions in mortality rates associated with intensivist-model ICUs ranged from 15% to 60%. On the basis of the most conservative estimate of effectiveness (15% reduction), full implementation of intensivist-model ICUs would save approximately 53, 850 lives each year in the United States."[6]

Reporting Systems

Voluntary Reporting

Many of the new publicly reported databases are considered voluntary. Yet, hospitals that choose not to report to voluntary databases may realize significant disadvantages.

One disadvantage stems from insurance company pressure. For example, a hospital might be invited to voluntarily report outcomes on its orthopedic surgery patients. It may choose not to report, and a key insurance company might say, "In the future, we will not contract with your hospital unless you participate in this publicly reported database." If the insurance payer is a vital contract for the hospital, then the hospital will most likely choose to participate.

An additional pressure hospitals receive is the use of data for comparison with that of other hospitals. On occasion, companies that collect voluntary data have released data to local news sources and published it on their Web sites. When data from four out of five hospitals within a community are published, then the fifth hospital feels the pressure of exclusion. The hospital's absence from the database may imply that the hospital is hiding something, or that its care is inferior to that of the other hospitals. This often persuades the hospital to participate in voluntary reporting in the future. Increasingly, both of these pressures are being used to increase voluntary reporting.

Hospital Licenses and Reportable Events

State departments of health are responsible for licensing health care facilities. Licensing is a stringent process. States have title regulations or codes that outline in detail the requirements for licensing. The state regulations expect health care facilities to be in compliance with all standards at all times.

In many states, state-licensed facilities are required to report unusual occurrences or adverse events. The language is written in such a way that hospitals can interpret what to report based on the degree of patient harm. Often, states levy large fines on health care organizations when they report adverse events, and this is a deterrent for health care facilities to report every error. Because fines can start in the tens of thousands of dollars, this is a significant issue for hospitals struggling with financial institutions.

Two forms of penalties are sanctioned by state regulations. Deficiencies reflect deficient practices and require immediate plans of correction. Citations are much more serious and require extensive and immediate corrections. The citations are what incur fines. Significant harm or unexpected deaths often result in citations.

Tip

Search for the Department of Health or the Department of Public Health in your state for the requirements related to hospitals' reporting of adverse events.

When an adverse event occurs, the health care facility's administrators must determine if the event constitutes a "reportable event" to the state. Each state describes these events. However, there is room for interpretation. Some state definitions are listed here:

California: Catastrophic or unusual occurrences that threaten the health, welfare, or safety of the patient.[7]

Florida: Life-threatening situations, serious adverse events described as wrongful deaths, brain injury, wrong limb removed, wrong surgery.[8]

New York: An unintended adverse and undesirable development in an individual patient's condition occurring in the hospital.[9]

Many facilities choose to self-report because if the event is reported by a third party such as a patient, the state investigation often results in more serious deficiencies or citations. The approach by states is punitive in nature and appears to do little to improve or overhaul flawed systems.

Mandatory Medication-Error Reporting

North Carolina was one of the first states to mandate reporting of serious medication errors to the state pharmacy board. Other states are attempting to implement similar laws.[10] Currently, California requires all pharmacies to have a quality-assurance plan in place that outlines the process for tracking and reporting medication errors. Other states have implemented some form of mandatory reporting of medication errors, but the exact definition of a serious medication error is still open to interpretation.

BABY JOSE

An Example of a Reportable Event

Little Jose was just two months old when his parents noticed he seemed to be getting progressively weaker. They took him to a hospital for treatment. The diagnosis shocked them: Jose had a heart defect. Though the problem had not been discovered at birth, as the baby aged, fluid had begun to form around his heart.

The doctor treating little Jose wanted him to have digoxin, a drug that slows and strengthens the heart muscle. Jose's doctor talked with the resident caring for Jose and explained the calculation for digoxin. Together, the doctors calculated the dose in micrograms for Jose's weight and then converted the dose into milligrams.

The resident started to write the order on Jose's chart when he was interrupted by a phone call. It was his attorney, who wanted to discuss some issues related to the resident's pending divorce. When the resident returned, he wrote an order for 0.9 milligrams of digoxin. The order was faxed to the hospital's busy pharmacy. The pharmacist thought the dose was too high, so he set the faxed order aside and paged the resident.

Later in the evening, the original order arrived in the pharmacy. The pharmacy technician put 0.9 milligrams of digoxin together with the order for the pharmacist to check. The pharmacist quickly looked at the digoxin with the order for 0.9 milligrams, not recognizing this was the same order he had questioned earlier. The resident had never returned his call because he had left the hospital and turned his pager off.

The nurse taking care of Jose received the digoxin from the pharmacy and questioned the order. She checked with another nurse, who was busy attending to other patients, and a different resident. The resident calculated the formula and came up with 0.09 milligrams. However, when he looked between his calculator and the vial, he missed one of the zeros.

The nurse infused the digoxin into Jose's IV line. Shortly after the infusion—as he was drinking his bottle—Jose began to vomit. The nurse recognized the complications and ran for the antidote to counteract the digoxin, but the baby went into cardiac arrest and died.[11]

Miscalculations; missing zeros; confusion between the abbreviations gm, gr, mg, mcg, mEq, ml, and cc; and transcription mistakes are significant contributors to medication errors.

Until technology systems can be implemented and are proven to stop errors, hospitals may benefit from sharing with one another their experiences with regard to medical errors. Yet, based on the JCAHO sentinel event data in chapter 5, it is clear that adverse events are underreported. Hence, solutions to prevent errors such as the one that led to baby Jose's death are not shared throughout U.S. hospitals rapidly enough.

Voluntary Medical Error Reporting

There are multiple benefits for reporting medication errors and sharing trend data between hospitals. The most critical of these are learning from the root causes of errors discovered during investigations and implementing proven safety strategies of prevention. Almost all hospital medication errors have the potential to happen within any hospital, and sharing proven safety strategies may reduce other errors.

The United States Pharmacopeia

The United States Pharmacopeia (USP) is an organization committed to the improvement of medication practices. It "promotes the public health by establishing state-of-the-art standards to ensure the quality of medicines and other health care technologies."[12] The USP receives data from hospitals with the aim of reducing and helping to prevent medication errors. The data are analyzed and returned to the hospitals to help professionals improve patient safety.

Medication Error Reporting (MER)

In 1991, the USP purchased the medication error reporting (MER) system from the Institute of Safe Medication Practices (ISMP). MER accepts error reports from clinicians and health care workers. Patients and consumers can call the organization; however, it is designed primarily for health care professionals. MER is voluntary and confidential.

Forms are provided to clinicians; the reports can be sent by fax or via the Internet. The ISMP and USP evaluate the data and create alerts on their Web sites. They share the data results with pharmaceutical companies and with the federal Food and Drug Administration (FDA). Medication labeling and packaging changes have occurred as a result of data from MER.

Tip

Call the United States Pharmacopeia (USP) at 1-800-23-ERROR (37767) to report a concern related to medication safety.

MEDMARX

In 1998, MEDMARX was created by USP in order to expand to an anonymous online medication error reporting database designed specifically for hospitals. MEDMARX allows hospitals to submit data with the goal of helping to identify and prevent medication errors. MEDMARX provides a root cause analysis template that feeds information back to the hospital in order to make improvements related to specific reviews. The hospital can pull its own trend reports to use to improve quality and enhance patient safety. Employees can report adverse events, either electronically or on paper, to be entered by a designated hospital pharmacist who has access to MEDMARX. It is a voluntary program.[13]

Tip

The USP also helps to standardize dietary supplements and medicines used in veterinary medicine. Log on to http://www.usp.org.

The Institute for Safe Medication Practices

"The Institute for Safe Medication Practices is a nonprofit organization that works closely with healthcare practitioners and institutions, regulatory agencies, professional organizations and the pharmaceutical industry to provide education about adverse drug events and their prevention. . . . ISMP is dedicated to the safe use of medications through improvements in drug distribution, naming, packaging, labeling, and delivery system design. This organization has established a national advisory board of practitioners to assist in problem solving."[14] The ISMP publishes alerts to help educate professionals regarding potential medication errors.

Tips

To learn more about the Institute for Safe Medication Practices, log on to http://www.ismp.org/.

ISMP publishes a consumer newsletter (see patient safety resources in appendix 2). Log on to http://www.ismp.org/ConsumerArticles/Issues/premier.pdf.

Findings from Voluntary Reporting Data

Voluntary reporting has been helpful in identifying problem areas in improving patient safety. The USP's fourth annual report, released in November 2003 and reflecting data from MEDMARX, found that more than one-third of hospital medication errors that reached the patient involved people age 65 and older. Fifty-five percent of fatal medication errors involved people age 65 and older.[15]

The data taken from the 2002 MEDMARX database reflected 192,477 medication errors. Of those errors, 3,213 resulted in patient injury. Errors of omission represented 43 percent of the total number of errors; wrong dosages, 18 percent; and nonauthorized drug errors, 11 percent. When harm occurred to seniors, 9.6 percent of the errors were prescribing errors. Hospitals reported that multiple factors, including complex systems and workplace distractions, played a significant role in contributing to medication errors.

Although these data highlight areas in which hospitals can begin to focus their efforts for improvement, the scope is limited because the reporting is voluntary. The data likely reflect some but not all of the troublesome areas related to medication use that patients are exposed to within hospitals.

Moving toward Solutions

The problem of medical errors does have solutions. Hospitals are implementing multiple programs as they strive to make changes. Many databases are making a difference; still, only a few of these are available to the public.

Consequently, too much information and data can also cause problems, such as where a consumer should look for answers when there are multiple data sources, some of which contradict each other. Hospitals produce such a large amount of data that information overload occurs, sometimes at the price of knowledge. The value of maintaining databases, which involves collection, analysis, internal reporting, and resource utilization, has to be questioned. If the data were more focused, centralized, and meaningful, perhaps patient safety improvements would occur faster. What is needed is not greater quantities of data, but data that are reliable and useful with regard to patient safety.

Public access to individual physician data is not feasible because of the blame factor and the high risk of litigation. Individual patient cases and physician-specific actions still need confidential protection. Conversely, other safety data need to become available to the public. This concept will be discussed further in chapter 12. The information released to the consumer must be standardized, reliable, and valid. Consumers need a basic understanding of data, but data must also be put in logical and understandable terms, much like the data that are used for consumer product reviews. (Additionally, this concept is also discussed further in chapter 12.)

CHAPTER 7

RAPID ADVANCEMENTS IN MEDICINE

Even admitting to the full extent the great value of the hospital improvements in recent years, a vast deal of the suffering and some, at least, of the mortality in these establishments are avoidable.

—Florence Nightingale, 1863

Keeping Up with Technology

Falling behind in the execution of continual safe medical practices has not been intentional behavior by the health care industry; rather, it is a casualty of massive expansion. As the industry has evolved, it has struggled to maintain suitable standards with regard to patient safety. Expanding hospital facilities, increasing knowledge base, growth in the number of professional disciplines, the technology boom, and the explosive growth of pharmaceuticals have revolutionized the practice of medicine.

Structural Growth

The first hospital buildings were simplistic in design, often built to house the infirm and dying. The Physick House in Philadelphia was the first hospital in the United States. The 32-room structure was originally built as a residence in 1786 by Henry Hill, a wealthy businessman. Hill lived in the house until he died of yellow fever in 1798. The house remained in the Hill family until it was purchased by Abigail Physick in 1815, who later deeded the home to her brother Philip. Philip Sygn Physick, a physician, eventually turned the house into a hospital. Dr. Physick worked hard to fight yellow fever. Dr. Physick went on to become known as "the father of surgery."[1]

Hospital growth has advanced a long way over the last two centuries—from former homes to the multilevel structures built in the 1940s to today's extremely complex campuses. In the days when structures were simple and communication was direct, it was easier to avoid errors.

Hospitals are frequently "landlocked," because initially the size and location of a hospital building was determined by the needs of the community at the time of construction. As the community grew, however, the hospital had to keep pace, even though there was little or no room for expansion. Often, hospitals have not been financially able to change locations and build new facilities. As a result, many hospitals have undergone years of adding on to structures—perhaps a new radiology department on the east side of the building, a new surgical suite on the north side, or a new intensive-care wing replacing one of the parking lots. Because of the multiple additions, the flow of patients becomes a challenge, promoting duplication and handoffs and exposing the patients to potential errors.

Growth of Medical Knowledge

Dr. Mark Chassim, one of the leaders in the patient safety movement, explains that in 1966 approximately 100 medical journal articles were published each year; by 1995 that number had grown to over 10,000.[2] This massive expansion of knowledge creates a challenge for each practitioner to keep up with the latest medicines, research, and treatments. In many of the leading specialties such as surgery, cardiology, and oncology, medical advances have evolved at an exponential rate.

Use of good continuing medical education programs, national conferences, peer review, and specialized journals help to focus clinicians. Nevertheless, each physician and health care professional must stay current to the developing changes within his or her specialty. Hospitals promote ongoing education, and professionals must stay diligent in learning the new advancements.

Professional and Specialty Growth

Many years ago, there were simply doctors and nurses. Nurses attended training programs, learning primarily within hospitals and clinics. Physicians attended four years of medical school, followed by specialized training.

Just how many specialties and disciplines are there in mainstream medicine today? Among physicians, refer to the board certification specialty list in chapter 4. Among nurses, there are various levels of nurses with different expertise, and there are numerous other clinicians as well. See chart on health care professionals at the end of this chapter.

Tip

Ask the name and title of all the health care workers who are caring for you. If someone is not wearing a name badge, ask him or her to please wear it when working with you.

Pharmaceutical and Technology Growth

The changes in medicine that have had the greatest impact on patients are the expansion of the pharmaceutical industry and the growth in technology. In general, both these industries have had an extremely positive impact on health services. The growth has been so rapid, however, that it is difficult to plan for all the potential dangers associated with them, specifically the scores of interacting components in both technology and pharmaceuticals. In addition, the burden on human practitioners to keep pace with the expansion in both trades bears an impact on the potential for medical errors.

Keeping Pace

A 73-year-old woman took an accidental overdose of Prozac when her pharmacist dispensed the wrong medicine in one of her other prescription bottles. He had filled two prescriptions for the woman, one for Prozac and the other for Restoril. He placed the Prozac in the Restoril bottle and the Restoril in the Prozac bottle. The pharmacist later said that he fills 800 prescriptions a day, an average of one prescription every 2.1 minutes.

Lay these time factors on top of handwritten prescriptions, look-alike medications and packaging, drug names that sound almost identical, and constant interruptions, and errors will occur. The probability of human error is tremendous in a system this large and complex.

There are now more than 11,000 prescription-grade medicines approved and produced for the consumer market. Thousands, perhaps even hundreds of thousands, more over-the-counter medicines, herbs, vitamins, and supplements are also readily available. All of these products have a potential for adverse drug interactions in patients.

In addition, the number of prescriptions being written is rapidly increasing. In 1990, approximately 1.8 billion prescriptions were written. In 2003, estimates were projected that prescriptions would more than double, reaching four billion per year nationally.[3] With such rapid growth in pharmaceuticals, the potential for many medications to look or sound alike increases. Listed here are just a few examples.

Antivert, Axert
Cefzil, Ceftin
Celebrex, Celexa, Cerebyx
chlorpropamide, chlorpromazine
Coumadin, Comtan
Lanoxin, Lovenox
Lasix, Losec
Lente, Lantus
Paxil, Plavix
Reminyl, Remeron
Serzone, Seroquel
Toradil, Toradol
Virilon, Verelan
Zantac, Zyrtec
Zocor, Zoloft

The confusion between chlorpropamide and chlorpromazine may have resulted in the death of a woman in New Jersey. According to Charles McLaughlin, his mother, Helen, became listless and was rushed to the hospital after taking the wrong medicine. Chlorpropamide is a diabetes medicine and chlorpromazine is a tranquilizer. Helen was supposed to get the tranquilizer. Instead, she received the diabetes medication, which lowers blood sugar. She later died. McLaughlin filed legal charges against the pharmacy.

A 37-year-old woman received a drug called loxapine, an antipsychotic, instead of her prescribed medicine, doxepin, an antidepressant. She thought her regular medicine had been replaced with a generic brand. After taking the wrong medicine, she suffered disorientation and a desire to commit suicide.

Tips

When receiving a prescription drug, open the medicine bottle and inspect the contents at the pharmacy. If the medication is different from your usual medication, immediately ask your pharmacy to recheck the medicine and make sure the order is correct.

DO NOT assume that a change in the way your medication looks is a substituted generic brand. Always confirm the change with your pharmacist. If after doing so you are still unsure, call your doctor.

Name Confusion

A young woman in labor in an obstetrics unit received an epidural anesthesia. Her blood pressure dropped, so the nurse called the anesthesiologist and received a verbal order for ephedrine 10-milligram through her IV. The nurse mistook the order for epinephrine and administered the medication.

The patient immediately developed a dangerously fast heart rate, her blood pressure soared, and she developed fluid in her lungs. She was treated and successfully delivered her baby.

The drugs ephedrine and epinephrine not only look similar when they are written, but they also sound similar when they are spoken.[4]

Dosing Differences

Verbal confusion, various accents, and the rapid exchange of information contribute to misinterpretations of medications. Many physician orders are given by telephone (known as TOs, or telephone orders). Nurses take these orders and then transcribe them to paper. The order is usually carried out before the doctor arrives. This process can result in misinterpretations or mistakes as described previously. Given the volume of medicines on the market, pharmaceutical companies face a growing challenge to use distinctive packaging for each medication. The industry has been helpful in changing packaging when issues have been brought to its attention, but because of the quantity of medications and the number of different manufacturers, it is nearly impossible to plan for and avoid all similarities. The Institute for Safe Medication Practices has led and continues to lead the efforts by issuing hazard alerts for hospitals and pharmacies as discussed earlier.

Consumers can help with this effort as well by reporting look-alike packaging as well as confusing and similar medicine names, labels, and directions. Report such issues to a pharmacist or to the FDA. See pictures shown in this book.

Tip

If you notice any look-alike packaging, pills, or medicines, contact the FDA at 1-888-INFO-FDA (1-888-463-6332). Also inform your pharmacist.

Advances in Technology

Innovations in health technology have revolutionized the industry. Microchip technology, telecommunication products, computer interfaces, sophisticated software, advanced monitoring systems, e-products, computerized surgery, smart IV pumps, gene research, precision implant devices, electronic transfer of radiology studies, and other advances have all served to promote patient care. Even so, multifactorial layering of these advancements poses problems in safety because of volume exchange of information and the potential for communication breakdowns, as illustrated earlier.

Anesthesia Safety, Industry Leaders

A medical discipline that has made some of the greatest advances in the arena of patient safety is anesthesiology. In years past, medical errors such as overdoses of chloroform and ether and poor airway management were prevalent in the administration of anesthesia.[5] Today, although the technology within the practice has grown exponentially, this specialty leads the way in striving to improve patient safety.

Between 1950 and 1970, anesthesia mortality studies showed that the death rate from anesthesia was approximately 1 per 10,000 patients administered anesthesia. The years between 1975 and 1985 saw a crisis in medical liability insurance for anesthesiologists. Premiums for practitioners within this specialty were six times the base rate for all other practitioners.[6]

In 1984, the Anesthesia Patient Safety Foundation (APSF) was established. The organization has implemented multiple practices to standardize and improve safety for surgical and procedural patients undergoing anesthesia. APSF states its mission as the following: "This Corporation is to ensure that no patient shall be harmed by anesthesia."[7] The practices APSF promotes include protocols for safe anesthesia procedures, standardization of anesthesia equipment, adoption of safety practice standards, simulation training in airway management, and advancing the knowledge base for practitioners of anesthesia. One study showed that at present, the death rate from anesthesia has fallen dramatically, to one in one million.[8]

Long before the Institute of Medicine released its report "To Err Is Human," the focus of many national and international anesthesiology conferences was patient safety, including preventing nerve and compression damage during prolonged surgeries. Back in 1989, the anesthesiology profession instituted the use of tutorials on patient safety for new anesthesiology residents. Included in these tutorials was "an overview of the specialty; preanesthetic evaluation and medication; technical details about anesthetic set-ups; the anatomy of the anesthetic equipment and its appendages; airway management (including endotracheal intubation); a sequence of assigned reading and/or advice about when, where, and what to study; bold print talks about anesthetic agents; and intraoperative monitoring."[9]

The APSF and the professional societies within the practice of anesthesia continue to focus on safety in their discipline. The standard the profession has set serves as a role model for other disciplines in the health care industry.

Tips

Log on to http://www.gasnet.org/societies/apsf/index.php to learn more about patient safety and anesthesia.

Before undergoing surgery, ask to speak or meet with your anesthesiologist to discuss the items that follow in this list.

Make a list of your anesthesia history. Include the items discussed in the following anesthesia tips. Share the list with the anesthesiologist each time you have a procedure or surgery. In the event that you undergo emergency surgery, have the list available for a family member to give to the anesthesiologist or surgeon.

Tell your anesthesiologist and surgeon about any allergies you have. Make a printed list of your allergies and give it to them.

If you have undergone surgery before and have become nauseated or vomited after the procedure, let your anesthesiologist know about this. He or she may be able to treat you with a medication to decrease these effects.

Tell your anesthesiologist and your surgeon about all the medications and over-the-counter products you take, including supplements, herbs, alcohol, minerals, and vitamins. Some of these products can affect your surgery; for example, ginseng can increase bleeding.

Figure 7.1
Health Care Professionals

NURSING	Registered Nurse	Licensed Vocational (Practical) Nurse	Pharmacist	Respiratory Therapy	Radiology Technologist	Laboratory Technologist	Paramedic & Emergency Medical Technician	Physical Therapist	Occupational Therapist	Physician's Assistant	Ortho Technician
Education	Associate to doctoral degree	One year of vocational training plus college prerequisites	Bachelor to doctoral degree	One to five years; registered or certified in specialized vocational training	Two to four years	Bachelor's degree; postgraduate degrees	EMT 1-3 and EMT; paramedic clinical and field training. Many paramedics programs result in associate degrees	Bachelor's degree; postgraduate degrees available	Bachelor's degree; postgraduate degrees available	Associate's to master's degree	Vocational program
License	State board with two-year renewals	State board with two-year renewals	State board and license	40 states now require state license	Certified	Registered or licensed depending on state requirement	Certified; registered with the National Register of EMTs	Passing the national certification exam results in a registered PT	Passing the national certification exam results in a registered OT	State certification with two-year annuals and six-year reexamination	

	Advanced Practice Nurse	Certified Nurse Aide	Pharmacist Technician	Respiratory Technician	Radiology Technician	Laboratory Technician		Physical Therapist Assistant	Occupational Therapist Assistant		
Education	Clinical Nurse Specialist, Advanced Clinical Nurse, and Nurse Educator receive additional advanced training and/or mentorship	90-100 hour course	May require a certificate	Vocational school	Vocational School	Vocational school or an associate degree		Two-year program; some states require a certification exam	Two-year program; some states require a certification exam		

	Nurse Practitioner
Education	Advanced practice nurses with additional graduate training who have the ability to diagnose patients and prescribe orders. They can have select specialties such as Emergency Medicine and Obstetrics

You may be positioned in various ways during surgery. If you have any preexisting injuries or illnesses, alert your anesthesiologist so that he or she can be more careful with those areas during surgery. For example, if you have nerve compression problems in your shoulder, the anesthesiologist can be extra careful with that part of your body.

If you are undergoing a surgery that will place you on your side or facedown, such as head, neck, shoulder, hip, leg, or back surgery, and you have a previous eye injury or eye disease, tell your anesthesiologist. Anesthesiologists take great care to protect your eyes and face during surgery, but it is imperative to give the anesthesiologist your complete medical history.

Ask what type of anesthesia you will be receiving. Write down the name. If you undergo the anesthesia well, you will want to let future anesthesiologists know what has worked well for you. In addition, if you have had an adverse reaction to an anesthesia product in the past, you will want to inform the anesthesiologist each time you undergo surgery.

If you have a history of injuries, illnesses, or diseases involving the mouth, teeth, nose, or throat, tell your anesthesiologist. This is important with regard to placement of the breathing tube.

If you have a history of difficult intravenous (IV) starts, let the anesthesiologist know before surgery.

Pediatric Anesthesia

Although the anesthesia specialty has taken a leadership role in use of safer anesthesia for adults, there are still further advancements to be made in the management of pediatric anesthesia. Many anesthesiologists who practice on adults prefer not to administer anesthesia to children. Pediatric airway management is unique, medications act differently in children as compared to adults, and the general body functions of the pediatric patient have to be distinctively managed. The practice of pediatric anesthesia is a subset and specialty in itself and takes an experienced specialist.

GRANT

A Specialized Need

In 1999, in a California hospital, two-month-old Grant Wray needed a repair of a hernia that was discovered after birth. It was expected to be a routine procedure. He was taken to the operating room. The operating room staff prepared Grant and a breathing tube was placed in his airway.

At the start of the operation, Grant's heart rate began to fall rapidly, and he went into cardiac arrest. In the hospital waiting room, Grant's parents heard an overhead page for a code pink (an emergency resuscitation on a child). They did not yet relate the code to their son, but they were concerned.

When Grant's mother saw three physicians walking toward her, she thought she had lost her son. The doctors explained the situation—they had almost lost Grant but were able to successfully revive him.

A later investigation revealed that the breathing tube used on Grant was too small. This caused a significant decrease of oxygen that ultimately led to his cardiac arrest.

Because of Grant's case and another serious case that occurred eight months later, when a child died from poor anesthesia management, the anesthesiologists wrote to the hospital administration and asked that the hospital either move pediatric surgeries to another hospital or bring in a specialized pediatric anesthesiologist. The anesthesiologists were not comfortable working with children, nor did they feel they performed enough pediatric cases to stay competent in this specialized practice.

Although concerned about losing the pediatric surgery population, the hospital administrators took steps to improve the practice of anesthesiology for children. They first required that a neonatologist be on hand during surgeries performed on infants aged one month or younger. They requested that the anesthesiologists evaluate pediatric patients well in advance of the surgery to discover whether they felt competent to manage that child. If not, the surgery would be performed elsewhere with a competent pediatric anesthesiologist. In addition, between 2000 and 2002, the hospital reduced the number of pediatric surgeries it performed by half. It also brought in a pediatric anesthesiologist to help handle the case load.[10]

A national task force on pediatric anesthesia has completed practice recommendations for the administration of anesthesia in children. These recommendations include the establishment of credentialing criteria for hospitals that provide elective surgery for infants and children. A brochure is available online at http://www.asahq.org/clinical/PediatricAnesthesia.pdf.

Tips

If your child is undergoing surgery, ask if there are anesthesiologists on staff who specialize in pediatric surgery. If not, why not?

Well before the operation, ask the anesthesiologist who will be performing the anesthesia on your child how many pediatric surgeries he or she performs per year.

Review the tips for adult anesthesia, and go over them with the anesthesiologist who will be working with your child during the surgery.

If you are uncomfortable with the anesthesiologist and his or her experience with pediatric cases, discuss this situation thoroughly with your surgeon and communicate your concerns. You may be able to choose another hospital that specializes in children's care.

Keeping Safety at the Forefront of Health Care Advances

There is no question that advancements in medicine have saved many lives, and there is no doubt that the expansion of the pharmaceutical industry has significantly increased the quality of life for countless individuals. People are living longer and functioning better due to advancements in technology and medicine. Nevertheless, continued focused attention on patient safety and the reduction of medical errors is the paramount goal for all the manufacturers as well as the entire health care community. Consumers can help prevent medical errors by identifying and reporting dangerous warning signs in medical products, technology, and medications.

Just as consumer product safety has improved because the public has taken the responsibility of reporting problems and applying pressure to the manufacturers, health services and hospitals can also learn and benefit from public input to enhance safety.

CHAPTER 8

OLD DESIGNS, PRONE TO ERRORS: SYSTEM FAILURES AND HUMAN FACTORS

Fallibility is part of the human condition
We can't change the human condition
We can change the system under which people work.

James Reason[1]

Although vulnerable communication systems are central to the dilemma, the crisis of patient harm goes beyond this. Fallible processes, fear of blame, fragmented human interactions, lack of practice simulations, and a sense of "this is just the way it is" result in widespread ignorance of the warning signs about the dangers that lurk within the health care industry.

The aviation industry provides a contrast. The public was starkly aware of the rash of airline accidents that occurred in the 1970s and 1980s. There was public, media, and governmental pressure to get to the root cause of the accidents and make commercial flights safer. In 1998 not a single fatality resulted from a commercial airline crash.

The U.S. health care system does not experience an airline crash–type disaster every few months. On the contrary, its events are more frequent. Deaths occurring in hospitals across the United States add up to the equivalent of a fatal airline crash every day.

Looking at the IOM's report "To Err Is Human," between 120 and 268 people die each day in U.S. hospitals (44,000 to 98,000 divided by

365 days). In order to draw this conclusion, the deaths stated in the IOM report are spread across the approximate number of U.S. hospitals—about 5,000. Each hospital in the United States kills 9 to 20 people a year by medical error, or one person every two to six weeks. Half of these deaths are preventable.

As the fatalities are diluted down by facility to a death every few weeks, the numbers are much easier to conceal than a plane crash. The public generally has little knowledge of these deaths. For physicians and essentially an entire industry that vows to "do no harm," it is time for this to change. Physicians, hospital employees, and other health care professionals are struggling with the dilemma. Individually, they each see few of the total number of people harmed or killed. The professionals and workers are isolated within small areas. When they do witness an unexpected, preventable death or injury, they talk among themselves about the appalling and shocking circumstances surrounding the death. They rarely ever take the event outside of the organization because of the code of silence that prevails. However, they remember the event and can describe it in detail for years afterward. Yet, they chalk it up to "the way things are" or "it's too bad these things happen; someone should fix the problem" or even "I knew that was a problem; I knew something was going to go wrong."

BABY GIANNI

In February 2002, Gianni Vargas was born in a New York hospital with a congenital heart defect. He had to undergo surgery during the first days of his life.

After surgery, at six days old, he needed potassium chloride to help his heart function better. In the neonatal intensive care unit, an injection was prepared and given to baby Gianni. Shortly after the injection the baby's heart stopped. Gianni could not be revived.

Baby Gianni was given a 10-fold overdose of potassium. Instead of 3.5 mil equivalent (mEq) of potassium, he was given 35 mEq. This volume of potassium chloride in an infant paralyzes the heart muscle.

What Was Learned?

The most shocking part of this tragedy is that seven years earlier, in the same hospital, in the same neonatal intensive care unit, a baby girl named Petra received a 10-fold overdose of morphine. She went into respiratory arrest; fortunately, she was resuscitated and survived the mistake.

A net of blame was cast in the event with Petra. The reaction by the hospital and the state department of health services to the error was to cast individual blame on the doctor and the nurse: "It was the inexperienced nurse's fault, it was the mistake of the intern who wrote the wrong order." One of the hospital's solutions was to implement a disciplinary policy against any physician who wrote a wrong order and did not correct it within 30 minutes.

Why did the intern write the wrong order? Why did the inexperienced nurse administer the morphine? What processes were in place that did not signal an alert and prevent the administration of the overdose of morphine? What system failed and resulted in the death of Gianni Vargas? Obviously baby Gianni was treated by a different doctor and nurse than treated Petra, but the same vulnerable hospital processes existed that allowed for these catastrophes. The same system failed both babies. Are those systems still in place? What about other neonatal intensive care units across the United States? What did hospitals share with each other about the error that affected Petra? What will be learned and shared about Gianni's death?[2]

Deaths and injuries are traumatic at any hospital, and it is often easier to look for individual blame, to target the person at the active end of the error, than it is to analyze and change a flawed system. Latent conditions are not easy to recognize prospectively, and often the processes involved in the error are fiscally challenging to change. Casting blame without targeting improvements in failed systems will only deepen the abyss of concealment.

MIGUEL

A Cascade of Failures

Miguel Sanchez was born in a Colorado hospital in mid-October. He was a healthy, seven-pound baby. The Sanchezes, who spoke only Spanish, had three other beautiful children, and Miguel was their welcomed new son.

As the staff was looking through the hospital records, they found that Miguel's mother had a history of syphilis. The staff was concerned that if the mother's syphilis had not been treated, it might be transferred to little Miguel. The nurses in the unit called the neonatologist.

The doctor ordered a laboratory test on Miguel for the syphilis, but the results would not be back until after Miguel and his mother had been discharged. The doctor was concerned that if the baby tested positive for syphilis,

Miguel might not get the follow-up treatment he needed. The doctor elected to treat Miguel.

The neonatologist consulted with a doctor who specialized in infectious diseases. The infection specialist recommended additional laboratory work and a spinal tap to check Miguel's spinal fluid for signs of infection. It was discovered that the day before, another neonatologist had performed a spinal tap. Though the result of the spinal tap was not yet available, infection could not be ruled out, and the neonatologist had already written an order for Miguel to be treated with penicillin.

The nurses were not familiar with penicillin treatments for newborn syphilis, so they wanted to confirm the appropriate medication. (There are many types of penicillin, so errors can occur with this drug.) The nurses called the health department and spoke with another infection specialist. The nurse handwrote a note for the penicillin order next to where the doctors wrote their orders. The nurse did not write the details of the order as is done with most telephone orders.

She wrote, "Penicillin G 50,000 units/kg." Miguel weighed a little over three kilograms (about 6 1/2 pounds). The nurse did not write the route of administration, nor the actual type of penicillin, which was penicillin benzathine.

The first neonatologist, who had performed the spinal tap the previous day, had handwritten an order for "Pen G 150,000 u IM" (the abbreviation IM stands for intramuscularly, an injection into the leg muscle of the baby; u represents units). The dose of 150,000 would match Miguel's weight. Above the order was the word benzathine. Typically, the order was written "penicillin G benzathine"; hence, the doctor's order was unusual.

The hospital pharmacist was consulted. Because this was not a routine treatment within the hospital, the pharmacist checked with two resources to confirm the correct drug amount and route. First, she checked the health department information, and then she verified it with information from another medication book. However, she misread the amount as 500,000 instead of 50,000 units. It was not unusual to give penicillin in hundreds of thousands and million-unit ranges. In addition, the handwriting on the physician's order was not clear; the pharmacist may have misread the 150,000 units as 1,500,000 units. The "u" symbol on the first doctor's order was not clear and looked very much like two zeros.

The pharmacist entered the order in the computer as 1,500,000 units. The computer issued no warnings about the maximum amount of penicillin for the weight of a baby. The pharmacist mixed the medicines in two syringes. In each syringe, the pharmacist mixed 1,200,000 units of penicillin in two milliliters of liquid. The total dose was now 2,400,000. The pharmacist put a bright green sticker on the syringe and clearly marked that only one full syringe and a fourth of the other syringe should be administered. Giving this amount (1 1/4 of the syringes) would total 1,500,000 units of penicillin. After mixing the medicine, the pharmacist noticed that one of the penicillin mixtures had expired, so she needed to replace the penicillin with another

Miguel's order.

mixture. Another pharmacy staff member gave the second penicillin mixture to the pharmacist, not checking the original order beforehand.

The nurses on the unit received the medicines from the pharmacy. Other than a green label stating to only give 1 1/4 of the medication, there were no other warnings on the syringes. The nurses wanted to be sure they were giving the medicines correctly, so the nurse taking care of Miguel and a nurse practitioner looked in another drug book. The book stated to treat the baby's syphilis with "Pen G Benzathine." The book did not warn against giving the medicine intravenously. Miguel's nurse was concerned that the amount in the syringes would cause Miguel to have an injection of 2.5 milliliters of liquid. She knew that newborns were to receive only a maximum of 0.5 milliliters of fluid in each leg. Two other nurses looked in another drug book to see if the medicine could be given intravenously to avoid the injection in the muscles. The medication book said that it was okay to give penicillin G very slowly through the IV. The book did not specifically mention penicillin benzathine, nor was there a warning against intravenous injection. The nurse practitioner checked yet another book, but penicillin benzathine was not mentioned.

The nurse practitioner assumed that benzathine was the brand name for the penicillin G. Because the order had been written oddly, the order seemed to confirm what the nurse practitioner was assuming. She concluded that the penicillin G benzathine could be given intravenously because it was the same as penicillin G. Indeed, it was not. In addition, the hospital policies were not clear, and her nursing license allowed her to alter physician orders when she determined that a different type of care was more appropriate for the patient.

The nurse caring for Miguel began to administer the medication in Miguel's IV. She slowly gave the medicine, thinking she was preventing Miguel the pain of having multiple injections in his legs. After she administered three-fourths of the medicine, little Miguel became unresponsive. Shock and dread filled the air as nurses and doctors tried desperately to revive Miguel. Their efforts were futile; little Miguel died.[3]

More than 50 System Breakdowns

A later analysis of the case of baby Miguel revealed that more than 50 system failures led to this devastating error. Some of those failures are outlined here, along with recommendations to prevent future such occurrences:

1. Several years before this incident, the mother had been treated for syphilis. Therefore, it was never necessary to treat Miguel. However, no written or electronic information about the mother's outpatient treatments was available on the baby's chart.

   Communication between the physicians' offices in written form or an electronic medical record now available could have held this information, averting the need to treat Miguel.

2. The mother's obstetrician had already evaluated the history of syphilis in Miguel's mother during the prenatal period and knew the mother had been previously treated. This evaluation was also not in the baby's record.

   Bring copies of your prenatal records when going to the hospital. Obtain the records from your doctor.

3. Language was a barrier.

   Mandate the use of translators. In Miguel's case, translators were available, but they were not used. A simple conversation with the mom may have negated the need to treat Miguel. Many hospitals and regulations now require translators to be present for discussion regarding consent and treatment.

4. The neonatologist was concerned about the mother not following up after she and her baby were discharged.

   Provide two-way communication to the mother's obstetrician and the hospital staff so that the obstetrician can address any unresolved issues at the postpartum follow-up.

   Also, improve health literacy by providing better educational opportunities for patients like Miguel's mother so they know to follow up and can communicate their medical history to other health care providers.

5. No rapid syphilis laboratory results were available for Miguel.

   Provide more rapid results and decrease turnaround times for lab tests. If a syphilis test result had been available, then a decision would have been made not to treat Miguel.

6. The hospital staff did not have experience with treating syphilis in newborns.

   Unless treatment is an emergency, do not allow staff to implement unfamiliar treatments without on-site supervision by an experienced professional.

7. No pediatric pharmacist was on staff at the hospital.

Hospitals that provide obstetric and pediatric services should have a pediatric pharmacist available. They can use one of the following three options:

a. Employ a pediatric pharmacist.

b. Provide a thorough pediatric internship for one of the current staff pharmacists.

c. For small hospitals, implement either a call system to a larger hospital with a pediatric pharmacist on staff or an on-call system to consult a pediatric pharmacist. A pediatric pharmacist would have recognized that pen G benzathine was not to be given intravenously, and that the volume and units of medication were too high both for an intramuscular injection and for an infant.

8. The second pharmacy staff member did not recheck the penicillin with the original order.

Mandate second checks with original orders whenever refilling medication orders. This double check could have picked up the overdose.

9. The multiple types of penicillin are confusing. Penicillin benzathine and penicillin G procaine should never be given intravenously. Yet penicillin G potassium and penicillin G sodium can be administered via an IV.

Clearly describe the different medications and the differences between them, as well as the proper route of administration for each, in all drug resources.

10. Clearly mark all warnings on the medications themselves about the appropriate route of administration. Make warnings large and visible. A small warning appeared on the manufacturer's syringe to give pen G benzathine only intramuscularly, but the warning was hard to read. The design of the syringe caused part of the warning to be covered. In addition, an electronic medical record could have predesignated warnings regarding the route of administration.

Additional high-risk processes and system flaws included the following:

1. The use of a handwritten order.

2. No clear policy on limiting the administration of unusual medications or treatments in the newborn without the presence of an experienced clinician skilled in that particular practice.

3. The use of varied and confusing drug resource books and information, with no specific newborn medication resource outlining the administration of penicillin.

4. The lack of preselected amounts (unit dose) of penicillin in the crystal form so as to avoid the need for complicated calculations and mixtures.

5. The lack of electronic communication between the health department and the hospital so that any advice is transferred via computer or other typed method instead of verbally.

6. No clear policy for altering physicians' orders by other disciplines. There was apparent confusion about this practice with the nurse practitioner.

Any enhancement or combination of enhancements in the system processes might have prevented this deadly error.

The most important issue was that there was no communication to Miguel's mother or father regarding the medication that was going to be given to their infant. Parents must always be the hub of any treatment provided to their children, despite the barriers that exist.

Criminal?

A wide net of blame was cast in this case. The three nurses taking care of Miguel were brought up on criminal charges of negligent homicide, the first time ever in the United States that nurses were criminally charged for an unintentional medication error.

One of the nurses went to trial; the other two entered pleas in exchange for reduced sentences. The nurse who went to trial was acquitted after the Institute for Safe Medication Practices presented an extensive analysis of the more than 50 system failures that occurred leading up to this error. The fact that Miguel died was tragic. The fact that nurses were criminally charged and paid extensive personal, financial, emotional, and essentially punitive prices for being caught up in a fragmented health system is also tragic.

The Newborn

Provided here is a list of tips for parents who will be in the hospital to have a baby. Remember that these are only guidelines; parents should check with their doctors and hospital before receiving any care. Please refer to the disclaimer at the beginning of the book.

Tips

If you speak a language other than English, insist on the use of a translator. It is your right.

It is important to become familiar with the routine at the hospital where you will be delivering your baby. Visit the labor and delivery areas before your baby is born.

Keep your own medical history about your pregnancies, including numbers of babies, types of labor, complications, and dates. Briefly summarize any illnesses or injuries you have had. Obtain copies of your prenatal records from your obstetrician and bring them with you to the hospital.

Ask if your hospital has a pediatric pharmacist on staff. Is one available for consultation? If not, why not?

Talk to and get to know the nurses who will be caring for your baby and ask to be involved in any treatment options that may be provided to your baby.

Once your baby is born, ask what will be done while you and your baby are in the hospital. What is the routine?

When you are admitted, insist on being informed of any medications or treatments that your newborn might need.

If an unusual treatment or medication is required for your baby, ask to be fully informed before care is administered. You can refuse the treatment until you have talked with another physician or experienced professional.

If any treatment is required, ask for written information about it.

The Blame Game and Human Factors

The Robert Wood Johnson foundation conducted a survey that showed 95 percent of physicians have witnessed a "serious" medical error.[4] Another recent survey, completed by Stanford University's Center for Health Care Policy and Center for Primary Care and Outcomes Research, surveyed 6,312 employees from 15 California hospitals. Thirty-nine percent of those surveyed reported they had witnessed a coworker do something that appeared to be "unsafe patient care," and 8 percent admitted that in the last year "they had done something that was not safe for the patient." However, "an identified common perception of 'fear of punishment' and 'lack of reward' for identifying and making mistakes existed." The study also found that a substantial number of unsafe acts in hospitals were caused by production pressures and other factors. In addition, a discrepancy existed between senior management views of progress on improving patient safety versus staff views of safety improvements. Senior management appears to think that patient safety improvements are moving farther along than the frontline workers believe is true.[5]

Targeting blame toward individuals promotes hiding errors and near misses because they fear punishment and retaliation. Before the tragic error occurred that killed Miguel, what if another nurse had almost made a similar type of medication error but never reported it? What if that nurse had been afraid to report the near miss because of fear of punishment? What if reporting other near misses could have saved Miguel? We may never know the answer to these questions, but hospitals need to create an environment that allows clinicians and health care workers to report all errors and near misses without the fear of retribution. It will be critical for leaders and regulatory agencies to move away from punishing employees. Otherwise, open disclosure of mistakes will move slowly, and not much will change on the horizon of medical errors.

Humans Are Not Perfect, So Change the Systems

Doctors and employees bring personal problems to work, become fatigued, misunderstand information, and perform multiple tasks at any given time. These human factors influence performance. People do make mistakes. Environments need to be evaluated for safety and improved to reduce human factors that lead to error.

Hospital systems should be redesigned to take into consideration the human factors involved in error analyses. James Reason's statement about fallibility is a starting point for understanding the human frailties and moving toward smoothing fragmented systems to reduce errors.

As we look at Miguel's case and consider other medical errors that have been reviewed, we must ask questions. How many other physician orders did the pharmacist have to fill when she was preparing Miguel's medicine? Was there a cardiac arrest that the pharmacist had to respond to in the hospital while she was filling Miguel's order? Was she the only pharmacist working at that time? Another pharmacy staff member was working, but he was a technician, not a pharmacist. How many other patients did Miguel's nurse have to care for? How many infant deliveries occurred that required the nurses to attend to other newborn babies during the time they were preparing Miguel's medication? How many previous shifts had the nurses worked in the days preceding the error? What kind of busy day did the neonatologist have?

Perhaps not all of these factors played into the medication error with Miguel, but the environmental issues listed here are routine in hospital settings.

Tips

Watch for overfatigued clinicians. If you sense a clinician is overtired and he or she is administering a medication, you can ask another clinician to check the medication for accuracy.

If a medication appears unusual, request that both a nurse and a pharmacist review the medicine.

Ask if your hospital has a safe medication practice pharmacist on staff whose sole purpose is preventing errors and improving the medication process. If not, why not?

Recognition of Human Factors

Human factors play a key role in all industries. The majority of people attempt to function well within their workplaces, but even good intentions can be spoiled by vulnerable processes. Pilots make errors. Nevertheless, if aviation pointed only to pilots as the root cause of airline accidents and expected that "stellar performance" and "pilot perfection" would prevent airline accidents, then flying might still be as dangerous as it was in earlier decades.

Aviation discovered that at least 70 percent of all accidents were rooted in system failures. Aviation leaders made a commitment to change. Whether the overriding concern was the industry's financial stability, nonetheless it was a commitment to reduce airline accidents and improve aviation safety.

In studying accidents, aviation looked at the human factors of pilots and air traffic controllers in great detail, all of which contributed to huge steps in aviation safety. Aviation went beyond the human factors with these professionals and included all members of this team. The industry did this almost two decades ago, as outlined here. This is a good example to be used in health care.

There are plenty of other clear-cut modern-day examples of the contributions of maintenance and inspection to aircraft accidents. One of the most spectacular was the Aloha Airlines accident in Hawaii on April 28, 1988. In this event, the forward upper fuselage of the aircraft separated in-flight from a point near the floor line. Passengers seated in this area were pummeled by slipstream and flailing structural wreckage, but through a combination of extreme good fortune and pilot skill, the airplane was landed with the unfortunate loss of one life, a flight attendant who was standing in the aisle at the moment the surrounding structure disintegrated. Subsequent investigation revealed that the airplane had been showing plenty of signs of impending structural failure, but these had been overlooked by the airline's maintenance staff [latent conditions].

Following the Aloha Airlines accident, the Office of Aviation Medicine (AAM) was tasked by the Offices of Airworthiness and Flight Standards to take a closer look at aircraft maintenance human factor issues. A review of human factors research revealed an almost total lack of information concerning the factors that affect the performance of aircraft maintenance technicians. Hundreds upon hundreds of studies and reports exist related to pilot and air traffic controller performance, but virtually nothing on mechanics and inspectors. This lack of research is somewhat puzzling, in view of the demonstrable fact that maintenance error can have just as devastating a result as pilot or air traffic controller error. The AAM research program has concluded that most human factors problems in aircraft maintenance belong to one or more of the following categories: 1. The worker, 2. The workplace, 3. Communication, 4. Training.[6]

In addition to the physicians and nurses, all other disciplines and health care workers should be involved in research methodologies to improve safety. "Human factors is defined as the study of interrelationships between humans, the tools they use and the environment in which they live and work."[7] Recognition of human factor engineering is a key step in reducing errors, but first, an understanding of how these factors play into medical errors is important.

The Human Factor of Fatigue

A landmark case involved the death of a young woman, Libby Zion, age 18, who entered a New York hospital with minor complaints of fever and an earache. The two medications prescribed for Libby, Demerol and Nardil, were not supposed to be taken simultaneously because of the strong possibility of an adverse interaction between them. Nevertheless, Libby received both medications, and for her, the combination was fatal.

The error was linked to an overworked and exhausted resident. Residents can work 60 to 130 hours a week, month after month, during their training. It was clear that the imposed human factor of fatigue was the root cause that resulted in Libby's death.

After news of this event spread, the public demanded reform. Following the Libby Zion case, New York was one of the few states to implement regulations limiting the hours residents worked. More recently, federal legislation was proposed to curtail training hours.[8] Still, almost two decades later, health care has not addressed many of the human factors that lead to errors. As of 2004, these regulations are not established; however, the Accreditation Council for Graduate Medical Education (ACGME) has created guidelines for limiting residents' work hours.

Lucian Leape, a pediatric surgeon and one of the authors of the Institute of Medicine report, stated: "Errors may occur because of interruption, fatigue, time pressure, anger, anxiety, fear or boredom. Work activities should not rely on weak aspects of human cognition such as short-term memory."[9] Dr. Leape's statement, "Systems that rely on error-free performance are doomed to fail," defines the need for health care leaders to use the techniques related to human factor engineering in aspects of system redesign. Leape further tells us that "the focus should be on prevention, not blame."

The Nuclear Power Industry

Nuclear power is a high-risk industry with strong potential for accidents and errors. In this industry, human factor engineering teams are integrated at the beginning of any major design process. These teams are the backbone of prospective planning to prevent accidents. This prospective planning and prevention may be one of the reasons that the nuclear industry's safety record surpasses that of health services. The importance of using human factor engineering in the nuclear power industry is stated in the following:

> The design resulting from the application of these methodologies, [prospective human factor planning, the use of human factor engineering teams, and human system interface] after its verification and validation, will enhance the plant operation's personnel performance when interfacing with the system and performing their tasks, this resulting in a decrease of the human error probabilities which will have a significant positive effect on the plant safety and availability.[10]

Teamwork

Doctors and health care professionals have worked wonders as they manage to function within problematic systems. In many ways, it is amazing that more errors do not occur, and the fact that they do not is a credit to the people in health care who work hard to prevent errors. Conversely, relying on human ability will, and does, eventually result in errors when the environment is fallible.

The acceptance of poor standards of communication, the lack of recognition of the human factors, and having to function within erratic health care systems has a stark effect on teamwork. Clinicians learn habits that allow them to get by. Workers respond in different ways to compensate for these current systems. Some professionals rely heavily on other team members, looking for a knowledgeable mentor to confide in and follow. Others may try to "fix" the problems with isolated solutions, and still others may pull away from these flawed processes and rely on independent thinking in order to cope within the chaos. All of these coping mechanisms deflect from functional teamwork.

Crew Management

Eglin Air Force Base in Florida created a process called Medical Team Communication. It was modeled after Crew Resource Management, a program that began in the 1970s and teaches pilots how to rely more effectively on teamwork.

According to author Fred Stone,[11] Crew Resource Management teaches flyers the principles of teamwork, communication, stress management, and other human factors to prevent aviation mishaps. The mission of Medical Team Communication is to create a safer patient care environment. The ultimate focus of this practice is to keep the patient at the hub of care and continually and consistently keep all the team members informed of changes in and departures from standards of care.

Tip

While in the hospital, ask who your team members are—their names, titles, and functions. This knowledge can assist you in asking the correct person directly when you need something, decreasing reliance on other people to pass your request to the right person. If you understand your team members' roles, you can often expedite their responses.

Situational Simulations

The Institute of Medicine defines simulation as follows:

A training and feedback method in which learners practice tasks and processes in life-like circumstances using models or virtual reality with feedback from observers, other team members and video cameras to insist improvement of skills.[12]

For several decades, the airline industry has utilized cockpit simulation training for pilots to practice urgent and emergency aircraft conditions. Health care has instituted simulation in a few areas, such as the practice of advanced life support (ALS), advanced cardiac life support (ACLS), and pediatric codes, as well as on a larger scale in disaster drills. In the ACLS practice, mannequins are used to simulate life-threatening heart abnormalities, and the learner must react using the American Heart Association's guidelines for treatment.

A simpler version of simulation practice takes place in cardiopulmonary resuscitation (CPR) classes that are offered in communities. CPR classes for health care workers and community members began in the mid-1970s and mimicked real-life situations of cardiac arrest. These practice situations were intended to diminish the panic that often develops during a crisis and to teach the learner the appropriate response to a cardiac arrest. There is no doubt that practices using these basic simulations have saved many lives.

The use of simulation is felt to be most beneficial in high-risk units, including intensive care units, operating rooms, and emergency departments. These rely the most heavily on efficient teamwork and accurate communication. Given that these areas pose the highest risk of error, with the administration of potent medications, specialized treatments, advanced technical equipment, and critically ill patients, simulation training is most certainly necessary.

The creation of simulation centers is increasing in the United States. These centers offer a range of simulated practices, including computer simulation, virtual reality training, computerized mannequins, and team simulations. Practitioners learn to place breathing tubes and catheters, perform colon and lung procedures, perform simulated surgery, and practice reacting to patient emergencies.

Several universities have implemented the practice of simulation. One early researcher in simulation training was David Gaba, who began a simulation center at the Veterans Affairs Hospital in Palo Alto, California, in 1995. At this center, a control room stands adjacent to the simulated operating room.

> From here, the instructor can call up and modify simulation scenarios, watch the performance of the simulation participants, direct the surgeon and nurses (actors), and even provide the patient's "voice" (through a speaker under the mannequin's head).... [A] critical part of simulator-based training is debriefing using the videotapes of the simulation session.[13]

The University of California at San Diego (UCSD), managed by the UCSD department of anesthesiology, has created the Center for Healthcare Simulation. The purpose of the center is to provide multidisciplinary, hands-on clinical education, training, performance, evaluation, and research using simulation-based training, patient safety research, and medical device evaluation.[14]

These lifelike practices allow clinicians to train for real-life situations. If mistakes are made, the practitioner can learn from the debriefing and error analysis and avoid making similar errors with real patients.

Equipment Failures

Dorothy Brenia, age 66, was in a hospital in Florida. Mrs. Brenia needed a medicine called nitroprusside to treat her extremely high blood pressure. The medicine had to be administered through an intravenous line. The nurse caring for Mrs. Brenia used the standard intravenous equipment available on the unit.

Unexpectedly, the nitroprusside rapidly infused into Mrs. Brenia's IV line. Mrs. Brenia's blood pressure dropped rapidly, and she went into respiratory arrest. She died two weeks later.[15]

Before 2003, there were few regulations regarding the type of IV pumps that hospitals used. In January 2003, the JCAHO mandated that accredited hospitals remove all "free-flowing" IV pumps, the type that resulted in Mrs. Brenia's death. Mrs. Brenia's accident occurred because an override clamp in the IV tubing failed to stop a free flow of medicine into her veins. Manufacturers of IV pumps have worked diligently to design new "smart pumps" that offer many protections against operator error. Aside from the pump, the tubing is designed so that no fluid will flow into the patient if the tubing becomes dislodged from the pump. The tubing design stops the flow of fluid. The smart pump concept is an example of prospectively using human factor engineering, in this case by the pump manufacturers, to make a fail-safe system. The nurse who cared for Mrs. Brenia turned in her nursing license, another casualty of broken systems and the blame factor.

Tips

Ask your hospital if it has removed all free-flowing IV pumps from its facility.

When receiving IV medications, ask what each medicine is for and the reason you are receiving it. You may receive multiple IV medications with more than one IV line. Ask the nurse to describe what medication is in each IV and what each medication is for.

When receiving IV medications, keep an eye on the area of your body into which the IV catheter is inserted. If the area becomes swollen, red, or warm, or any combination of these, alert your nurse immediately.

Medical Equipment

In 1990, the Safe Medical Device Act was implemented. This act requires that hospitals report to the Food and Drug Administration all events in which medical devices or equipment caused or may have caused a death or serious injury. Hospitals are provided tracking forms for these occurrences, and they often cross-reference the event on their incident report tracking forms. The FDA defines a reportable event as one that is "life threatening, results in permanent impairment of a patient's body structure or function, or needs any medical or surgical intervention to prevent permanent damage to a patient."[16]

Proactive Human Factors Designs in Equipment

Recently the U.S. FDA has focused attention on medical equipment. Many medical products may pose design flaws; they are diverse and confusing and can cause operator errors. Even when well-trained people are operating the devices, errors can be unintentionally built into products that may cause harm to patients.

The FDA's Office of Device Evaluation now requires human factor assessments on all approved medical devices. The FDA describes the benefits of human factor engineering (HFE) in the development of medical equipment:

- Reduced risk of device use error
- Better understanding of device status and operation
- Better understanding of a patient's current medical condition
- Easier-to-use (or more intuitive) devices
- Reduced need for training
- Reduced reliance on user manuals
- Easier-to-read controls and displays
- Safer connections between devices (i.e., power cords, leads, tubes, etc.)
- More effective alarms
- Easier repair and maintenance

The FDA states that HFE should take place early in the product-development process. It should include tools such as analysis of critical tasks, use of device hazard and risk analysis, and realistic use testing. Medical devices can sometimes harm patients, family members, or healthcare providers. The potential harm arises from three sources:

- Failure of the device
- Actions of the user (or use-related errors)
- Hazards associated with device use are a serious problem

A combination of influences leads to use-related errors with medical devices. These include:

- Medical devices can be complex;
- Medical devices are often used under stressful conditions;
- Users may think differently than device designers do;
- Consumers now use devices that were originally designed for experienced medical personnel; and
- People blame repeated use errors on the user, rather than on poor product design or inadequate instructions for use, so people don't recognize the need for human factors.[17]

Fail-Proof Barriers

The prospective use of HFE is limited within hospitals, yet human errors are embedded in most hospital activities. Proactively planning for these human fallibilities can help improve multiple health care system designs.

To use the example of aviation again, a key component of military aviation is to have no one point of failure. Backup systems exist wherever there is a chance for failure. If health care can create barriers without holes, then greater numbers of errors will most likely be avoided.

Tip

To view FDA safety alerts on medications and food, log on to http://www.fda.gov.

Another high-risk area for device problems is nuclear medicine. The Center for Devices and Radiological Health (CDRH) also recognizes that manufacturers must evaluate human factors at the beginning of the product-design process to prevent design flaws. The FDA and the CDRH programs are an excellent start to the integration of proper design into medical equipment systems. Much prospective planning, eliminating reliance on memory, reducing assumptions, and narrowing the opportunities for error are required with the new standards.

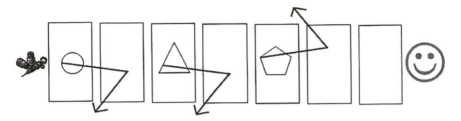

Fail-proof systems.

The Front Line

The front line of health care is engaged in a battle for patient safety. Old designs, multilayered communication systems, and disenfranchised health care professionals all carry tremendous responsibility in the war on medical errors. Most health professionals endeavor to improve patient safety, and numerous groups are working to strategize and reduce errors. Nonetheless, many of these strategies do not center enough on human factors, practice situations, crew management, and other methods that may reduce flaws in medical systems. Further research into these methodologies should substantially increase across hospitals and health systems.

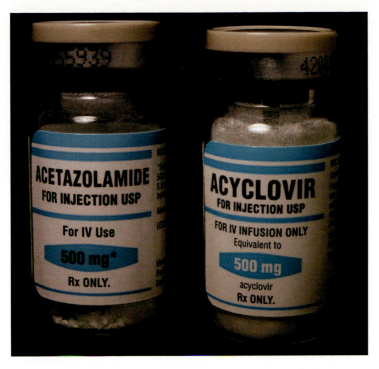

Too close for comfort. Two medications with significantly different uses:
Acetazolamide 500 mg, used to treat seizures and glaucoma; and Acyclovir
500 mg, used to treat severe forms of the herpes or shingles virus.

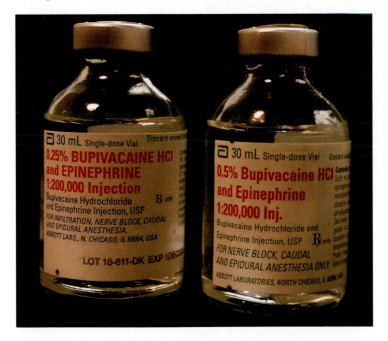

0.25% Bupivacaine HCL and 0.5% Bupivacaine HCL. Injectable anesthetics
used to block pain in the nerves. Two different doses packaged similarly.

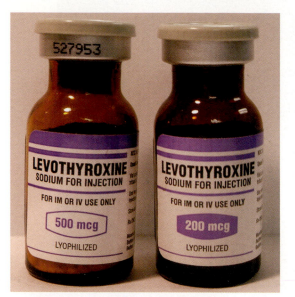

Levothyroxine (levoxine) 500 mcg and Levothyroxine 200 mcg. Confusion regarding labeling of this medication has resulted in multiple medication errors, including patient deaths. The FDA and the ISMP have issued alerts regarding this drug and labeling confusion. There has been confusion between "mcg" and "mg," confusion as to how the medication is mixed, and name confusion between a heart medication called lanoxin and levoxine.

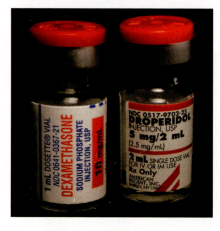

Droperidol 5mg/2ml and Dexamethasone 10mg/ml. These two drugs have very different uses: Droperidol is used to reduce nausea after surgery, and Dexamethasone reduces inflammation and can be used to reduce swelling after traumatic injuries, treat some types of cancer, and treat severe joint disease.

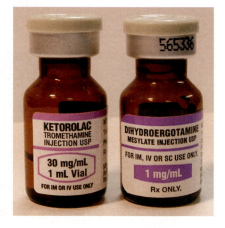

Similar packaging with different uses: Ketorolac (toradol), used to reduce inflammation and pain, often after a surgical procedure; and Dihydroergotamine, used to treat severe migraine or cluster headaches, and alters vascular blood flow to the brain.

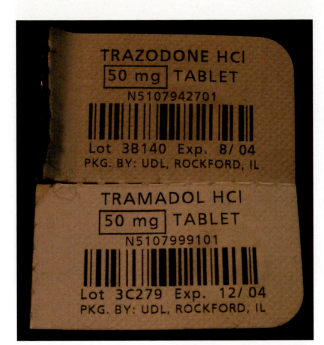

Almost identical, but look closely, they are different. These drugs have been mistaken for one another: Trazodone 50 mg, used to treat depression; and Tramadol 50 mg, used to treat pain.

Lisinopril 20 mg and Lisinopril 10 mg. The dose is different. This medication lowers blood pressure, therefore doubling the dose by mistake can result in a significant drop in blood pressure.

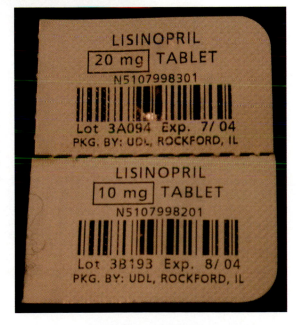

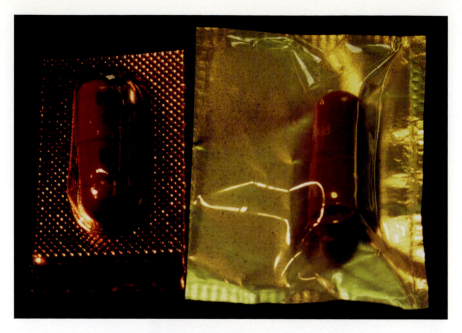

Rifabutin 150 mg and Rifampin 300 mg. Both are used as an antimycobacterial in HIV or Tuberculosis patients. They look the same, but the capsules are different strengths.

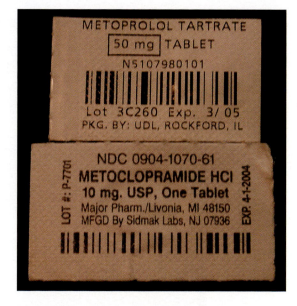

Metoprolol 50 mg, used to treat high blood pressure and chest pain, and Metoclopramide 10 mg, used to treat stomach disorders and nausea.

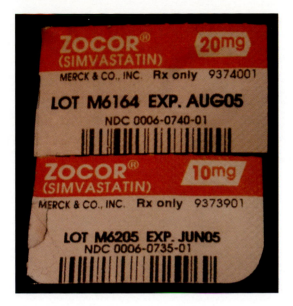

Zocor 20 mg and Zocor 10 mg, a cholesterol lowering medication. Different strengths, but identical packaging.

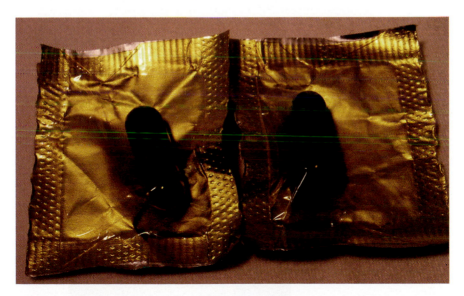

Duricef, an antibiotic, and Carbatrol, a strong medication used for seizure disorders.

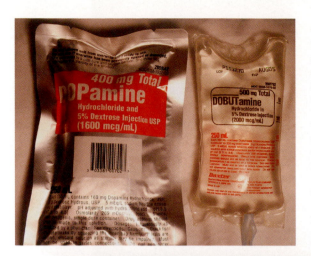

"Tall man" lettering is a new FDA recommended safety improvement standard. For example, DOPamine and DOBUTamine. Both of these are potent IV medications with similar names. These two medications have been mistaken for one another, causing patient harm. Both medications are used for the treatment of congestive heart failure and shock caused by the inability of the heart to function properly.

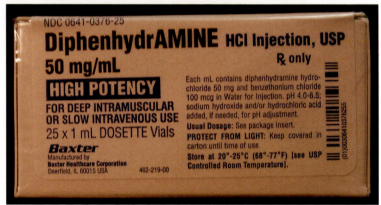

DiphenhydrAMINE. "Mine" and "mide" have been mistaken for one another.

BuPROPion instead of buPRIPion. The picture is of an antidepressant. The other, buPRIPion, is a medication that helps with smoking cessation.

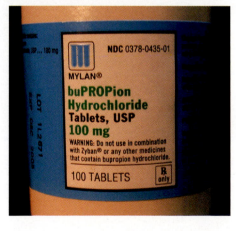

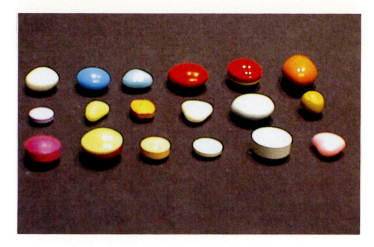

I. Can you tell which ones are pills and which ones are candy? Can your children? These average medications can be found in many households.

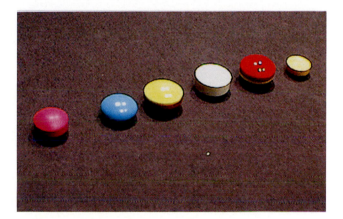

II. Pills or candy?

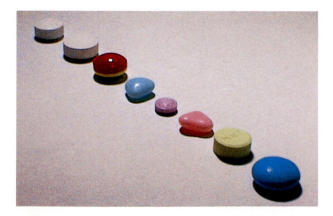

III. Pills or candy?

CHAPTER 9

DISCLOSURE

Evidence and examples support the fact that people who are victims of a medical error want information about the error, in detail and rapidly, after the event occurs. This early disclosure may help to offset litigation. Mistakes occur, but what angers people is the attempt to hide information afterward. The error affecting Ben Kolb, discussed in chapter one, was disclosed, and as horrible as the tragedy was, the family could begin to cope with the loss because they had an explanation.

DR. KARL SHIPMAN

To Disclose or Not to Disclose?

Dr. Karl Shipman was admitted to a Colorado hospital in September 1997 with a broken wrist. The healthy, active 64-year-old had fallen off a ladder. Dr. Shipman had practiced at the Colorado hospital as an internist and had formerly been the chief of medicine.

Dr. Shipman required surgery to repair his wrist. After the surgery, he began to develop problems with his wrist, and an infection set in. The infection spread to his spine, and he developed incapacitating pain. Two months after his fall from the ladder, Dr. Shipman died in the intensive care unit.[1] Dr. Shipman's daughter, Debra Malone, an intensive care unit nurse at another hospital, later stated, "He died from a broken wrist—in his own hospital... The hospital would not admit the error, apologize or address change." Malone eventually filed legal action against the hospital.[2]

In contrast to Dr. Shipman's case, Martin Memorial Hospital took steps to remedy systems and disclosed details regarding Ben Kolb's death. Hospital leaders made a full analysis, including a detailed investigation of all the steps and systems that led up to the fatal medical error. They immediately stopped all practices related to using these medications in the operating room, analyzed the syringes and their contents, evaluated the handoffs, and made significant changes to prevent future errors.

After completing the investigation surrounding the error, realizing that their systems had failed and that they were responsible, the hospital leaders elected to meet with the Kolb family and admit full responsibility for the error that led to Ben's death.

Dr. George McLain, the anesthesiologist who was called to help revive Ben after the error was made, stated, "The damage was already done, the child was dead, OK? So you have two choices. You can lie. You can cover up. You can spin it. Or you can be honest. And the nice thing about the truth—basically, [you] only have to tell it once."

McLain added, "You know, you look in a parent's eyes that you know their child is dead because of a mistake. And that, you know, it's, How could you take my baby away? Because you know, this was a very beautiful healthy child that should not have died."

Ben's mother could not even comprehend that this minor procedure took her son's life. She wanted to know when Ben would wake up. "Well, well, when can I give him his Christmas present? I bought him one, I want to give him the present today."

Tim Kolb, Ben's father, said, "I was in shock. I was in utter shock that such a simple mistake, number one, could occur in an operating room. And number two, that it could so easily take a life."

Disclosure discussions may not be able to occur immediately following a death because of shock, but they should occur fairly quickly after the event to clarify facts. As painful as it was to hear the facts about Ben's death, hearing those details is exactly what the Kolbs needed to begin understanding and dealing with the event.

"Revenge wasn't there for me," said Tim.

So on the list of things he wanted from the hospital, money was not at the top. People being fired was not at the top. "No, no," said Tim.

Was it just an answer? "Oh, yes," Tim responded. "We wanted to know what happened. We wanted the truth."[3]

Tips

Not only did Martin Memorial Hospital make a full disclosure about the error involving Ben Kolb's death, but the hospital also participated in creating a video to help teach other clinicians about the problem of medication errors. The award-winning video, *Beyond Blame*, is used in hospitals throughout the United States. The American Hospital Association distributes the video to its member hospitals. The short video covering Ben's story, *Beyond Blame*, is available through Bridge Medical, http://www.bridgemedical.com/beyond_blame.shtml.[4]

While you are in the hospital, if you feel that something has been done incorrectly, talk to your nurse or doctor. If the issue is not resolved, ask to speak to the nursing supervisor or manager.

While in the hospital, if you feel like you have tried to resolve an issue with your nursing manager, your physician, or both and the issue still seems unresolved, ask to speak with a patient-relations representative. The representative will complete a written report and follow up with you regarding the issue.

Disclosure

Disclosure is a term used in hospitals and in legal arenas to signify an unveiling of the facts related to an incident.

Five types of disclosure are discussed here:

1. Disclosure by a hospital to a patient about a medical error
2. Disclosure by a physician to a patient about a medical error
3. Disclosure to peers by an employee about committing a medical error
4. Disclosure to a supervisor by an employee about committing a medical error
5. Disclosure to a patient about a near miss

Disclosure to Patients

In some hospitals, the leaders strongly embrace disclosure to patients, and these hospitals have engaged in this practice for years. For most hospitals, though, the practice represents new territory. There are no hard data to quantify whether outright disclosure about injuries and deaths will result in reduced liability, but some of the early studies are promising.

Taking the First Step

Long before the release of the Institute of Medicine's report "To Err Is Human," the Veterans Affairs (VA) Medical Center in Lexington, Kentucky, changed its policy on disclosing errors to patients. In 1987, after losing two large lawsuits that totaled $1.5 million, the VA hospital moved to a practice of full disclosure surrounding medical errors.

The researchers Kraman and Hamm studied the practice of full disclosure at the Kentucky facility and concluded the following:

> Despite following a policy that seems to be designed to maximize malpractice claims, the Lexington facility's liability payments have been moderate and are comparable to those of similar facilities. We believe this is due in part to the fact that the facility honestly notifies patients of substandard care and offers timely, comprehensive help in filing claims; this diminishes the anger and desire for revenge that often motivate patients' litigation. In our experience, plaintiffs' attorneys, after first confirming the accuracy of the clinical information volunteered by the facility, are willing to negotiate a settlement on the basis of calculable monetary losses rather than on the potential for large judgments that contain a punitive element. This can benefit a facility by limiting settlement costs to reasonable amounts. It also fairly compensates patients who have been injured because of accident or error. This is important because such compensation is deserved, but is infrequently offered.[5]

This new practice was well received by hospital personnel. The proactive changes continued because hospital leadership and the staff felt this was "the right thing to do."

The hospital used a new approach to risk management, implementing the following policy on patient disclosure: "The medical center will inform the patient and/or the family, as appropriate, of the event, assure them that medical measures have been implemented, and that additional steps are being taken to minimize disability, death, inconvenience, or financial loss to the patient or family."[6] The Kentucky VA hospital became a role model for the entire VA system.

In 1995, the Department of Veterans Affairs rewrote the section of its policy manual that dealt with risk management policies; this material is now incorporated into a section titled "Patient Safety." Referring to patient injury caused by accidents or negligence, the new wording was taken directly from the Kentucky VA hospital's disclosure policy.[7]

The Veterans Affairs Process for Disclosure

The VA risk management committee performs an investigation and evaluation when an accident occurs. Three components are listed in the process for dealing with medical errors. The first is patient notification: "When the risk management committee identifies an instance of accident, possible negligence, or malpractice, it investigates the facts." Second, a meeting with the patient, the patient's family, or both is arranged by the hospital. The following occurs at the meeting:

> The subsequent meeting is with the chief of staff, the facility attorney, the quality manager, the quality management nurse, and sometimes the facility director. At the meeting, all of the details are provided as sensitively as possible, including the identities of persons involved in the incident (who are notified before the meeting). Emphasis is placed on the regret of the institution and the personnel involved and on any corrective action that was taken to prevent similar events.

> The committee offers to answer questions and may make an offer of restitution, which can involve subsequent corrective medical or surgical treatment, assistance with filing for service connection, . . . or monetary compensation. After the meeting, the patient, surrogate, or next of kin is assisted in filing any necessary forms and is given the names and numbers of contact persons who can answer any additional questions.[8]

Humanistic Risk Management

The VA was one of the first organizations to move toward humanistic risk management. Traditional risk management uses methods to track and prevent liability claims for hospitals. It attempts to defend against potential and actual litigation and often results in defensive stands against lawsuits; this often creates an adversarial relationship with patients and their families:

> Humanist risk management is an approach that responds to medical errors with several principles, including full disclosure and compensation as appropriate. Most importantly, the focus is to maintain a compassionate hospital and patient relationship, with a continued strong role as the patient's caretaker.[9]

From a financial and preventive standpoint, not enough evidence exists to say that full error disclosure to patients will reduce medical malpractice litigation. Nevertheless, the work in Kentucky and ultimately the policy the VA embraced on a national scale appears to be a significant step in the right direction.

The Veterans Affairs Patient Safety Leadership

Implementation of this policy by the VA was just one part of a massive overhaul of the agency's patient safety practices. In response to the IOM research, the VA implemented all of the recommendations from the IOM report that were applicable to its programs.

According to Dr. James Bagaian, director of the VA National Center for Patient Safety, new patient safety training, analysis, and reporting has been implemented at all 172 VA medical centers in the United States. Additionally, now when an error occurs, the involved clinician reports it and a team of medical experts from the National Aeronautics and Space Administration (NASA) analyze the error and make recommendations for prevention.

The VA has implemented the use of technologies including an electronic medical record. At the Washington, DC, facility an electronic medical record with embedded practice guidelines for physicians and bar coding for improved patient identification and medication matching is in place.[10]

Full Disclosure

What about the case of Mrs. Hoffmann, who received Remeron instead of Reminyl? Should the cardiologist disclose the error to Mrs. Hoffmann and her son? Can the incident of combativeness be attributed to a manifestation of her progressing Alzheimer's without her medicine? Is the hospital accountable for the additional $24,812 cost she incurred? The answers may seem simple; however, the combative incident might not have been related to the medication error. Perhaps the error could recur to Mrs. Hoffmann in the future if it were not disclosed.

Mrs. Hoffmann and the Resolution

Mrs. Hoffmann's case was resolved without litigation. A hospital executive, the cardiologist, and the hospital attorney met with Mrs. Hoffmann and her son. Hospital leaders reviewed the steps in the admitting process and how the medication mistake happened. They discussed how the staff misheard the word Reminyl because of Mrs. Hoffmann's heavy German accent. The leaders suggested to Mrs. Hoffmann that she keep a written list of her medications. They shared how the hospital had changed its admitting practice and that the primary physician's office would always fax the patient's medication to the admitting department before the patient arrived.

Two weeks after Mrs. Hoffmann was discharged from the hospital, the parties reached an agreement. The hospital leaders offered to pay the portion of Mrs. Hoffmann's medical bills that occurred after the cardiac procedure.

The agreement was expensive, yet probably far less costly than a lawsuit would have been. It would have been even more cost-effective to have a system in place that prevented this error.

Tips

Once you have left the hospital and you feel that you have an unresolved issue, write a letter to the hospital patient-relations department. State your concern, and stick directly to the facts. Number or bullet your concerns. Ask for a written response by a certain date, but allow two to three weeks so the hospital can investigate your issue.

If the written response does not address your concerns, ask for a meeting with a patient-relations representative, a hospital administrator, or both.

If you have a serious concern, call the hospital and ask to speak with one of the hospital executives. Before calling, write down your concerns so that you can discuss the issue with clarity.

One of your patient's rights is the ability to file a grievance. The hospital is obligated to assist you with filing a grievance with the state department of health if you elect to do so. Contact the hospital patient-relations department if you wish to file a grievance, or review the information on your admission paperwork for the phone number.

Hospital versus Physician Disclosure

Conflict arises when a hospital and physician become entangled in deciding who should take the blame for a medical error. The hospital might decide that it can accept the responsibility for a medical mistake, such as what occurred with Mrs. Hoffmann; however, the physician may not want to admit his or her part in the error.

On the other hand, a physician may elect to admit to an error, but hospital leaders may not want the liability or the financial responsibility of disclosure. These dilemmas do occur. Nonetheless, these predicaments focus on the "blame factor," not on working toward resolution for the patients or improving health systems.

The most critical factor is a dual approach, much like what was used at Martin Memorial Hospital. Yes, the surgeon injected the wrong drug, but the failed systems, wrought with latent conditions, set the situation up. The surgeon could have blamed the hospital for faulty procedures and poor quality control, and hospital leaders could have blamed the surgeon for not rechecking the medications before the injection. If this conflict had arisen, no one would have benefited, least of all the Kolbs. The family needed an explanation of the mistake. They needed answers, not concealment of the facts. In the case of Karl Shipman, perhaps Debbie Malone would have reacted differently if information about her father's death had been disclosed and dealt with more openly.

When disclosing events to the patient, it is imperative for the hospital leaders and the physician(s) to meet together and sort out the details and accountabilities of the error before the patient meeting. This patient meeting should occur only after a rapid and full investigation is completed, with the root causes identified and an action plan in place to correct and prevent comparable errors. Once the root cause analysis is completed, then responsibility can be sorted out more accurately. An initial meeting with all parties may be helpful to state the intent of disclosure and to inform the patient and family that an investigation is under way. Physicians and hospital leaders should be in agreement to any actions prior to a family meeting.

Patients who are not told the details surrounding an adverse event feel that there are missing links. Anger may be dispelled if the patient and family are informed and involved in action steps surrounding the medical error. Certainly, this type of involvement would enlighten the patient to the facts about the situation. Additionally, disclosure may clarify misinformation that can lead to anger, uncertainty, and ultimately litigation.

Fear

Unfortunately, because of fear of medical malpractice litigation, red marks in the National Practitioner Data Bank, and loss of well-established reputations, both physicians and hospitals can easily revert to cover-ups and casting blame. This fear is a driving force in health care as to why disclosure is not utilized more frequently.

Other Players in Disclosure

Casting blame does not occur only between administrators and doctors. Physicians cast blame on nurses and other health care professionals. The blame factor occurs between two nurses, doctors, or other clinicians as well as between the different physician specialists. Occasionally, these blame battles are charted in the patient's medical record.

The nurse caring for Mrs. Hoffmann documented the following in Mrs. Hoffmann's medical record: "The patient would have been okay if the doctor had not made the medication error." These types of notes are valuable for attorneys who may be looking for accountability, but they do little for resolution of the problem.

Hospitals, physicians, and clinicians need to develop a reasonable approach to disclosure that will benefit the patient and family. When a path of calamities occurs, it can be easy to point a finger at the various players involved in the care of the patient. This moves away from resolution for the patient.

Peer-to-Peer Disclosure

"We need to create a culture of safety in hospitals and other health care organizations, in which errors are openly discussed and studied so that solutions can be found and put in place," said Dr. Dennis O'Leary, president of the JCAHO.[11]

One of the most challenging areas that physicians, clinicians, and hospital staff face is the disclosure of an error to peers. Colleagues and other clinicians can come down hard on the person who made the error: "How could you have done that? What were you thinking?" Fear of losing the respect of peers as well as one's professional reputation is a significant factor that cannot be overlooked when a clinician is considering whether to admit to a medical error. Coworkers may have more compassion if they better understand latent conditions that put the professional in a vulnerable situation and led to an error.

Cover Up or Report?

There are no studies to quantify the number of medical or medication errors that are concealed or "fixed," but such events do occur. If a nurse administers a wrong medication with no ill effects, such as giving Tylenol to the wrong patient, would that nurse always file an incident report? Many certainly would, but some would not. They know that no harm was done.

Technically, administering any medication without a physician's order is a violation of a nurse's license, and as such it is a violation of hospital policies. Even so, this scenario is that of a nonharmful event. Nurses and other clinicians might tell a peer about the minor error such as the Tylenol administration. A peer may even agree with the person who made the error that they do not need to report it. After all, they reason, no harm was done. Some of these clinicians may tell the patient about the incident, but they may not formally report it.

However, making a more serious medical error, where the patient is harmed, is pure devastation. Negative pressure from peers can exacerbate the horror of a serious mistake.

Changes in attitude and acknowledgment of the impact that an error can have on a clinician may be helpful to the clinician's recovery. The person at the active end of the error needs to comprehend that they were at the end of a line of vulnerable processes, and they alone are not to blame. Learning together about holes in the barriers and uncovering latent conditions as a team are critical to error prevention.

Peer Challenges of a Blame-Free Culture

A survey done by the Institute for Safe Medication Practices found that 26 percent of staff nurses felt that if a nonpunitive practice were put into place, carelessness might increase. This study also found that the front line staff (22%) were more likely than administrators (16%) or managers (9%) to believe that a nonpunitive culture may be detrimental to an organization.

With regard to "bad apple" thinking, collectively nurses (19%), physicians (13%), and pharmacists (16%) agreed more readily than executives (10%) that a nonpunitive culture curtails the hospital's ability to get rid of the "bad apples."

Additionally, collectively, management (25%) and staff (18%) perceived that implementing a nonpunitive environment tolerates failure.[12]

Long Memories

In a hospital unit, when a patient is killed by a medical error, the event is deeply embedded in the memories of the clinicians and other workers. If the person who was at the sharp end of the error is not terminated and elects to stay employed at that hospital, then coworkers tend not to trust that person again. This mindset results in others wanting to suppress their own errors and near misses. No health care professional wants to become marked as a bad clinician. In reality, however, this type of peer pressure makes the environment even more dangerous and punitive.

Steps need to be implemented to teach peers supportive reactions to errors—reactions that will bring the clinician making the error "into the fold" in a caring manner. If recovery from errors is implemented in a sensitive way, professionals will most likely have less fear of being ostracized, and the chances that errors are brought to the surface early will most likely increase. In hospitals, if open discussion and resolution are to take place, the culture must change with regard to the ways people think, react, and function when an error occurs.

Utter Devastation

One night in a busy Nebraska hospital, the code team was summoned to treat a patient in cardiac arrest. Within a short time, another code was called. By the time the night was over, the code team had run from code to code providing CPR and advanced life support treatment to four patients.

On occasion within hospitals, two codes might occur in one night, and rarely three. It was extremely unusual to have four patients go into cardiac arrest within a short period. As the night unfolded, a pattern started to be revealed.

In the busy pharmacy, a pharmacist had filled four orders for mixtures of an antibiotic called metronidazole. That night, four patients throughout the hospital were scheduled to receive their doses of metronidazole. It was soon revealed that the four patients had received a drug called Mivacron instead of the metronidazole. Mivacron is a paralyzing drug that causes respiratory arrest.

The blame fell immediately on the pharmacist and the pharmacy technician working that night. Administration targeted them both for termination. As a more detailed investigation was completed, however, it was discovered that multiple misaligned processes had led up to the series of medication errors.

First, the medicines had identical packaging; they both came in tiny foil-wrapped packs with tiny printing. Second, the Mivacron in this type of packaging was new to the pharmacy, never having been stocked or used before. Third, the pharmacy staff had not been notified that this was a new product brought into the pharmacy. Fourth, the drugs were stored in close proximity to each other because of their alphabetical order. Fifth, there were not sufficient rechecks of the medicines once the mixtures got to the floors. The error got through the susceptible barriers, allowing a significant impact on four patients.

Two patients survived the medical error; the other two died.[13]

Needed Recovery Methods

When a critical error is made, the professional at the sharp end of the error is utterly devastated. Often, health care professionals have chosen their line of work because they desire to help people and to be an agent for healing. Frequently the person who made the error is his or her own worst enemy, asking repeatedly in despair, "How could I have done that; why didn't I check better?" The individual takes on the full responsibility that should be carried by the entire system. Many physicians and health care professionals never recover from being at the sharp end of a severe or fatal error.

Carrying the Blame

In a large inner-city hospital, Dr. Z, the on-call anesthesiologist, received an urgent page to come to the intensive care unit. A 54-year-old man, who had been admitted for a severe asthma attack and had started to recover, was now developing worsening asthma.

The patient was rapidly deteriorating and needed a breathing tube inserted. To assist with the intubation, the anesthesiologist administered 50 milligram of ketamine. The breathing tube was secured.

Within a few minutes of the intubation, the patient went into cardiac arrest. A code was called and the team worked to resuscitate the man, but they were unsuccessful.

A later investigation found that an overdose of ketamine had been accidentally administered to the patient, causing a fatal heart attack.

The anesthesiologist, who had participated in 12 surgeries that day and ran two previous codes within a few hours of this code, had given a twofold overdose of the drug. The emergency code cart stored vials containing different-strength doses of ketamine right next to each other. The labels were both red and white and looked almost identical. The printing of the doses was tiny and hard to see. Instead of grabbing the 50-milligrams-per-milliliter vial, he grabbed the 100-milligram-per-milliliter vial.

Dr. Z was completely devastated. The anesthesiologist, who had previously had a stellar record and was highly respected by his peers, took on the full responsibility for the mistake. This was his first serious medical error. The case was extensively peer reviewed and a full analysis was performed. Dr. Z's peers initially rallied around him, but support began to drop off over time. No counseling was offered to Dr. Z.

Over the next two years, Dr. Z fell into a deep depression; he attended fewer departmental meetings and social gatherings, and his appearance deteriorated. He started to become hostile. His marriage fell apart and a bitter divorce ensued. Eventually Dr. Z left the practice of medicine.

Physician Recovery from Error

Traditionally, few services are offered to physicians who make severe medical errors. The doctor is supposed to be above mistakes;

perfection has often been the standard for physicians. This deep-rooted tradition may put extreme guilt on a doctor who does make an error. Medical staffs lend some opportunity for support through physician well-being committees. However, the primary intent of these small, highly confidential committees, often headed by a psychiatrist, is to deal with substance abuse problems, such as alcohol or narcotic addiction, or personal behavior problems that spill over into the clinical setting. The groups' focus has not been error recovery. The medical executive committee usually mandates referrals to this group, and these referrals are sometimes viewed as embarrassing or a "red mark" against the doctor. Medical staffs offer few intercessory services to physicians to help them recover from grave medical errors.

Although it has not been studied, the physician who makes an error may benefit from being involved in the peer review process. When an error is serious, the physician is often brought before the peer review committee for input and to explain the circumstances surrounding the error. It can be difficult for a doctor to appear before a committee of peers and detail the event. Even so, when a physician can handle the experience without defensiveness and can treat it as a learning experience, it may be therapeutic. This is especially true when the peers show compassion and take steps toward resolution.

The peers have a unique insight to errors. The colleagues "walk the line" every day, and they know that given just the right circumstances and the correct cascade of misalignments, that any of them are just a moment away from making an error themselves.

Medical staffs should consider creating additional supportive measures—aside from peer review—that focus on physician recovery from medical errors. Error recovery is a new field in health care, and more research needs to be done. In the meantime, open discussions about errors and more supportive methods need to be developed.

Team Members

Government employers and many private organizations sponsor employee assistance programs (EAPs). According to the federal Office of Personnel Management, EAPs provide "free, confidential short term counseling to identify the employee's problem and, when appropriate, make a referral to an outside organization, facility, or program that can assist the employee in resolving his or her problem."[14] Hospital EAPs should consider the impact of medical errors on both individuals and team members. The devastation of hurting a patient can have equally distressing consequences on all team members. There may be an advantage to setting up team recovery support services. The impact of an error can result in acute unresolved grief. Strategies that allow individuals and teams to work through the grief may positively affect recovery. Recovery team intercession is a concept that needs further research and investigation in health care.

Some hospitals have started employee recovery programs through their employee assistance services to help employees work through the trauma of making a grave or fatal error. These programs attempt to take employees through the event and use principles of grief counseling. Programs such as these are a beginning; however, peers need help to react supportively when an error is made. Increased education on dealing with errors should be provided to professionals.

Disclosure to Supervisors

In an article referring to the error with Jesica Santillán the *Wall Street Journal* wrote, "Now, a movement is gaining ground that could transform medicine's culture of blame into a culture of safety. Its main tenet is to encourage voluntary disclosure of medical errors without fear of punishment."[15]

Since the IOM report and its emphasis on a blame-free environment, medical error disclosure by clinicians has gained a great deal of attention. The intent is to create a nonpunitive atmosphere where health care professionals can openly discuss errors, including disclosure to supervisors. Creating this setting encompasses a difficult culture change for health professionals. Clinical training, not just for doctors but also for nurses and other clinicians, has traditionally emphasized the importance of perfection: "The patient's life is in your hands, so you must never make an error." These deeply instilled values are difficult to change. Fear of reporting to a supervisor and the possibility of being reported to a regulatory or licensing board is overwhelming.

Health care leaders recognize the importance of a blame-free environment in theory; in spite of this, however, when these leaders begin to write policies, they leave in an "out" clause. With this clause, the health care institution reserves its right to fire someone who makes an error if they think the situation is serious enough to warrant such action. This clause essentially deflates the concept of a blame-free environment.

It is reasonable to leave language in the policies against drug and alcohol abuse, and certainly to deal with someone showing criminal intent to harm patients. Occasionally, these kinds of issues surface in hospitals, and such problems need to be dealt with firmly and swiftly. Termination, legal action, or a combination of the two are completely appropriate. However, the "out" clause that deals with a very serious error still blames the clinician or worker for the error and does not direct the blame toward bad systems.

Leaders have hung on to the "out" clause, reflecting back on egregious medical errors they witnessed. Horrific incidents are very difficult for leaders to forget. Clinical leaders find it particularly challenging to let go of such incidents because they cannot help but place themselves back into the patient care setting and ponder, "How could that nurse have made such a terrible error? *I* would never have done anything *that* bad!" These lingering memories will not easily disappear. The "out" clause issue needs more open discussion and research as the advancement of patient safety continues.

Occasionally, supervisors threaten employees who make errors by telling them they will face criminal charges for their actions. Again, this is the enculturation of being perfect or perhaps of supervisors believing they could never make an error of the same magnitude themselves. Additionally, the supervisors may simply not understand the components of system failures. In their view, their threats will scare employees so much that they will not make more errors. In reality, however, this approach causes all employees to further hide and conceal errors.

Sentinel Event Review Teams

Sentinel event review teams are a recent development in health care settings, and the more effective ones have attempted to be non-punitive in nature. They usually involve the front-line practitioner(s) at the active end of the error. Participating in the sentinel review experience can be intimidating even for a confident person, but if the team facilitator approaches the event in a blame-free manner, there may be benefit in being part of the investigation group. Even so, the focus of sentinel event teams is to establish the root causes for the error, not error recovery.

Traditionally, blame for errors is still deeply embedded within the medical setting. The Louisiana nurse who injected the concentrated potassium into Mr. L (refer to chapter 5) had her license suspended. Other nurses and clinicians have had their licenses revoked after a serious error that could be attributed to system failures instead of individual responsibility. Much more work needs to be done in this area.

A Near Miss

Ten years earlier, in the same emergency room where Debbie, the 14-year-old patient with diabetes (see the introduction to this book), almost received a 10-fold overdose of insulin, another near miss occurred that was quite similar.

A new emergency room nurse, who had transferred just a few weeks earlier from a medical floor to work in the ER, prepared a dose of fast-acting insulin to give to his patient. A standard nursing practice at the time required that nurses double-check insulin before administering the drugs. The new ER nurse drew up a dose of insulin and followed the standard practice for double-checking with another nurse.

He took the doctor's order and the insulin syringe to the second nurse. The second nurse immediately noted a serious error in the amount of insulin. The first nurse had drawn up 40 units of the fast-acting insulin instead of 4 units. As had occurred with Debbie's nurse, he had misread the small syringe markings. The nurse checking the order immediately identified the problem. The first nurse instantly recognized what *could have* happened and began to shake from fright at the thought of harming his patient with such a massive overdose. Most likely this nurse would never make the same error again. At that time, there was no format for reporting near misses. Yet, 10 years later, in the same busy emergency room, another nurse almost gave Debbie a 10-fold overdose of insulin. This time, the standard practice of double-checking high drug concentrations was not followed. The knowledgeable patient prevented the error.

If the near miss from 10 years earlier had been studied by the hospital and additional safety practices had been put in place, maybe Debbie's near miss could have been averted long before she had to intervene to stop the potential error. A medical error should never get this close to a patient; the patient should not have to be the last and final barrier. Even so, as systems exist now, the patient will need to be alert, knowledgeable, and hands-on in preventing errors in his or her care.

Tracking Near Misses

The term near miss has been used and accepted in aviation and is now being used in the health care industry. Some hospitals use other terms, such as "close call" or "never event."

Tracking near misses is a challenging task, though it may be one of the most crucial areas to study in health care. A number of hospitals have started to track near misses on incident reports, adding data fields to their incident report forms so they can evaluate the prevalence of these occurrences. Determining the circumstances surrounding the steps leading up to each near miss will help hospitals and researchers understand system vulnerabilities and human factors that interact and set the stage for errors.

Other Studies in Near Misses

Researchers at the University of Maryland are studying near misses with regard to traffic safety. Dr. Jeffrey Hadley is the principal investigator of a study at the National Study Center for Trauma and EMS at the University of Maryland School of Medicine. Dr. Hadley said,

> We want to know as much as possible about what was happening in the critical few seconds just before a crash or near-miss. By contrasting the information associated with these two types of incidents, the study will provide a new understanding of the human factors that are most important to avoiding an imminent collision. The study is the first to seek the specific circumstances surrounding a large number of near misses. It is estimated that the typical motorist experiences a hazardous driving situation every two hours on the road, and narrowly averts an accident about once a month.[16]

The Veterans Affairs Tracking of Close Calls

The Department of Veterans Affairs is a leader in the area of tracking and analyzing near misses. This agency uses the term *close call* to describe the occurrence. Dr. James Bagaian is helping to lead the project. He has worked with NASA in the study of space disasters.

"When you have a close call, you should look at it with every resource," Bagaian said. "Before, close calls made up well less than 1% of the events reported and analyzed [at the VA]. Now they make up 50 to 94% of all cases reported. If you normalize it for a full year, we're looking at a 900% increase in reporting."

That does not mean there are more close calls. "It means we are getting a better chance to look at things we couldn't look at before. It's a learning opportunity. The more reports, the better patient safety gets."[17]

The state of Florida has started a coalition to report near misses, using NASA's program as a model. The main goal of the coalition is to improve patient safety and ease the medical malpractice crisis. One of its key objectives is to create a reporting system for medical near misses so it can study the factors surrounding the events. The legislative plan is called "The Coalition to Heal Healthcare in Florida."[18]

Reporting Near Misses to Patients

Few, if any, near misses are disclosed to patients. One reason for this. is that often, not all the parties are aware of a near miss. A wrong medication might have been mixed in the pharmacy, but the medication error was caught and never got to the floor. The nurses and the patient would have no knowledge of this near miss. Even so, the pharmacist might track this error in order to avoid it in the future. In a case like this, there is no need to alarm the patient as long as future preventive steps are taken by the pharmacy.

Nonetheless, in a more significant near miss situation, it may benefit the health care team to report, analyze, and even involve the patient if an element of the near miss may have involved the patient. For example, if the surgical side marking was done incorrectly and the marking process involved the patient, then it may benefit the health care team to work with patients to improve the process.

A CLOSE CALL

In a busy hospital pharmacy a handwritten order came in for a patient on the obstetrics and gynecology unit for two grams of magnesium sulfate, used to decrease the frequency and force of labor contractions. The order was for a 37-year-old woman. The pharmacist mixed the medication and sent it to the floor. The nurse caring for the patient had left the floor to attend a hospital meeting and another nurse had taken over the woman's care. The second nurse had a patient who was requiring immediate help, so she asked yet another nurse to give the drug that had arrived on the floor.

The third nurse picked up the original order and the magnesium sulfate mixture. The nurse checked the woman's identification and prepared to administer the magnesium. "Tell me about your baby," the third nurse asked. The woman replied, "Oh, my baby is in high school and he plays basketball." Something clearly did not make sense to the nurse. "What are you in the hospital for?" The woman replied, "I have just had a hysterectomy." The nurse

---

Morphine or magnesium?

said, "Were you supposed to get morphine for your pain?" "Yes, as a matter of fact, I was about to ask about that."

The original order had been for two milligrams of morphine sulfate, not two grams of magnesium sulfate. The mix-up in these drugs occurred because the full names of the medications were not clearly written or typed out. This near miss happened to be caught by an observant nurse who suspected something was wrong.

Certainly, a 37-year-old hysterectomy patient on an obstetrics and gynecology unit could have been mistaken for a patient in labor. The woman was cold and well covered in blankets, lying on her left side, facing away from the nurse. The narrow escape was disclosed to the woman and her husband in detail, and the nurse took on the full responsibility and profusely apologized.

Systems could have been in place to stop this order from being written in this fashion. The name of the medication should have been fully written out and not abbreviated.

Table 9.1
Do Not Abbreviate

Morphine sulfate	MSO_4
Magnesium sulfate	$MgSO_4$

A Culture Change on Disclosure

Disclosure to patients regarding medical errors, supportive environments for those who make errors, and analyzing near misses represent new areas for the health care industry. In concept, these ideas are embraced; nonetheless, there remain many traditional fears associated with open discussion of medical errors. The health care industry still has high expectations of its clinicians, and this is not unreasonable if clinicians can practice in a safe environment with systems in place to avoid errors. Until a safety culture is established, limited disclosure and fear of retaliation for making an error will persist.

CHAPTER 10

BEYOND MEDICAL MALPRACTICE

MRS. S

Perspectives

On a Sunday in late April, Mrs. S, age 82, was admitted to a moderate-sized suburban hospital in Washington state. Mrs. S, who had been cared for at a residential facility in the community and had been mostly bedridden, now had developed breathing problems.

After the hospital team stabilized her breathing, a registered nurse did a full assessment of Mrs. S and noted a large, deep bedsore on her lower back. The nurse immediately repositioned Mrs. S so that no pressure would be on the sore. The nurse then paged the skin team and the physician. The skin team did a full evaluation of the bedsore, along with Mrs. S's risk for developing further skin breakdown.

Mrs. S was immediately put on a special mattress, and the latest and best skin treatments were started to help the wound heal. She was put on an IV antibiotic and her nutritional status was assessed and adjusted. The therapy department assisted her with small walks to strengthen her legs. Additionally, she was helped up to sit in a comfortable chair three times a day and was repositioned in her bed every one to two hours.

Mrs. S's daughter Jane, who lived in Connecticut, had been on a long business trip to Europe and could not get back to visit her mother until the following week. Mrs. S continued with her skin treatments and the bedsore started to heal, although the wound was still quite deep.

Jane and her husband, Jack, arrived at the hospital the following Friday. As Jane was greeting her mother, she noted the large sore on her mother's back. Jane became upset and asked the nurse about the bedsore. The nurse explained the skin treatments that Mrs. S was receiving. However, this nurse was unaware of Mrs. S's history and the fact that she had been admitted to the hospital with the bedsore. Mrs. S suffered from short-term memory loss, and all she could tell her daughter was that she got the sore "in this place."

From this information, Jane and her husband assumed that the bedsore had developed in the hospital. As a few days passed, Jane's anger increased about her mother's skin breakdown, even though Jane could see that the hospital staff was aggressively treating the bedsore.

Mrs. S's breathing problems subsided and her skin continued to heal nicely. Jane and her husband decided to move Mrs. S back to Connecticut to a nursing home near them.

Thirty days after Mrs. S was discharged, Jane hired an attorney to represent her mother. The attorney filed legal charges against the hospital for elder abuse and neglect. The information was sent immediately to the hospital's risk management department, and a full investigation was performed. Because of the misinformation and lack of clarification, Mrs. S's daughter, the hospital attorney, a nursing supervisor, a skin team member, and two administrators were tied up with legal matters surrounding Mrs. S's case for three months. It was finally discovered through the investigations that the hospital did not contribute to the bedsore, and in fact, it implemented state-of-the-art treatments that ultimately led to Mrs. S's full recovery.

The real culprit, the residential care facility, was not served legal papers until five months after Mrs. S left the city. Jane also filed a complaint with the state, which led to an investigation of the residential care facility. During the investigation, it was discovered that the facility clearly had significant issues of neglect and that in the five months during which the legal matters were tied up at the hospital, at least five other people at the residential care facility had developed significant bedsores, malnutrition, and dehydration.

Get the Facts

Immediately after an error or perceived error occurs, there is often uncertainty and anger. Because communication is inconsistent within hospitals, it is critical to look past the confusion and determine the facts regarding a perceived or actual error.

In the case of Mrs. S, there were clearly communication failures. When Jane arrived, the nurse caring for Mrs. S was from an outside nursing registry. The nurse was a good clinician, but she did not readily have information on the history of Mrs. S's skin breakdown. She could have read the patient's entire paper chart, but she was also caring for five other patients.

The doctor who admitted Mrs. S was not the same doctor who assumed her care during the time that Jane was visiting her mother. In addition, Mrs. S's daughter came to the hospital at times other than when the doctor came in to see patients, so they never spoke directly to each other. In addition, Jane had trouble getting through to the doctor's office because she attempted to call too early in the morning or during the lunch hour. She could reach only the doctor's answering service, which would not take a message because it was not an emergency. Misaligned communication systems made it difficult for all parties to receive correct information and clarify misunderstandings.

Litigation and Settlements

At times, litigation against providers of medical care may be necessary; however, lawsuits against physicians or hospitals can take an average of two years. Also, they are extremely costly, and the plaintiff may not win. Costs of judicial claims are difficult to track because most claims result in settlements, as opposed to being decided by a jury. Additionally, settlements may result in lower awards than jury verdicts.

Raging Debate

Currently, debate is raging over increasing physician malpractice insurance premiums, jury settlements, and amounts paid for noneconomic awards in malpractice suits. In January 2003, surgeons from West Virginia hospitals went on strike to protest the increasing costs of medical malpractice insurance premiums. In May 2003, in Chicago, more than 4,000 physicians marched at a rally to demand tort reform. At that rally, American Medical Association chair-elect William Plested III declared, "Preserve access to care" and "Will your doctor be there?" Protests from the doctors urged citizens to take note: "Wake up Chicago, wake up Illinois, wake up America . . . your health care is in crisis!"[1]

Premiums are rising substantially and exponentially for many specialties. Surgeons and obstetricians pay the highest premiums because of the risks involved in their specialties. Some surgeons pay as much as $73,000 per year, with expectations of premiums rising to $100,000 in 2004.[2]

Obstetricians have been hit hard by these rising premiums. Shelby L. Wilbourn, M.D., who is board certified in the practice of obstetrics and gynecology, testified before a joint hearing of Congress.[3] She stated that she had left a thriving practice in Nevada after 12 years because of the astronomical rise in insurance premiums. She told the hearing panel, "One obstetrician in Nevada was paying $141,760 per year, with a number of physician premiums rising 50 percent in just one year." She also stated that Nevada faced a crisis because of the dwindling number of physicians. She was concerned that the decreasing number of doctors would not cover the number of deliveries occurring each year.

In addition, it was recently reported that some obstetricians in Florida pay premiums as high as $210,000 a year. There are some key reasons that physicians who deliver babies pay such high premiums. First, they are at risk to manage difficult newborn deliveries with the potential for injury to the babies. In addition, the statute of limitations for damages that may occur at birth runs until the child is an adult. Technically, a child may reach school age before the parents claim the child has some injury or disability caused by birth trauma.

Besides Nevada and Florida, other states hit hard by increasing premiums include Arizona, Illinois, Texas, Massachusetts, Mississippi, Ohio, New York, Pennsylvania, and West Virginia. An increasing number of multimillion-dollar awards are being paid out by juries; the medical and insurance industries say this situation is affecting the rise in premiums. Published information on average jury award rates in the United States varies: the AMA quotes a source that states, "Nationally, median malpractice jury awards rose from $500,000 in 1995 to $800,000 in 1999."[4]

California Set the Stage

Three types of damages are assessed in malpractice awards: punitive (intended to punish), economic loss (considered actual damages such as medical bills and loss of income), and pain and suffering. In 1975, California legislators put a cap of $250,000 per claim on the amount that could be awarded for medical malpractice claims related to pain and suffering. California does not cap punitive or economic damages. Most physicians and medical associations and the insurance industry agree that legislation that limits award payments will serve to curtail the rising costs of insurance premiums. Numerous physicians from states that do not have such caps have moved their practices to states with settlement caps. Other doctors are retiring early, and a few physicians have even chosen to leave the practice of medicine.

Some states with limits on malpractice awards are New Mexico, Wisconsin, and Indiana. Debate over cap limits continues in many state legislative bodies. States including Florida, North Carolina, and Georgia have proposed legislation for reform. However, in late March 2003 Florida's senate overturned a bill to cap settlements.

According to the American Medical Association, premiums in California for physicians have risen 167 percent as compared to premium increases of 505 percent in other states.[5]

The Other Side

Some groups like the Foundation for Taxpayers and Consumer Rights, a consumer advocate group, argue that the true stabilization of premium rates in California came as a result of California proposition 103, which passed in 1988, and not from the cap limits on pain and suffering damages. Proposition 103 implemented insurance reform measures.[6]

Several studies conducted by universities and legal organizations with the support of citizen groups concluded that insurance premiums rise or fall because of swings in the economy. Some of the study results could not find a direct correlation between rising malpractice awards and higher premiums. A few results showed that in some cases the average amount awarded by juries had decreased while insurance premiums increased.[7]

Public Citizen, a consumer advocacy group that presents public viewpoints to Congress, argues that a historical pattern has been established by which insurance rates rise based on the investment market.

> Spikes in medical malpractice rates are temporary and due to investment losses and poor pricing policies by the insurance industry rather than a result of medical malpractice litigation. Because of these factors, double-digit premium rate increases are occurring in all insurance products in 2001 and 2002, as evidenced by the state-by-state analysis in the report. Medical malpractice claims have remained constant in recent years. Increases in malpractice awards have been far below the pace of medical inflation.[8]

However, some patients have had significant harm inflicted upon them from medical errors. Many of them argue that if you cap pain and suffering damages you will hurt vulnerable economic populations such as children, seniors, the unemployed, and people who are not the sole income providers for their family.

Linda's Story

Linda McDougal, who lost both breasts because of a pathology error and who subsequently suffered from severe infections at the operative sites, was not the sole income provider for her family. She testified before a congressional joint hearing on the subject of medical malpractice caps:

> The medical profession betrayed the trust I had in them. While there are no easy answers, apparently now the insurance industry is telling Congress it knows exactly how to fix what it believes to be the "problem" caused by malpractice—by limiting the rights of people, like me, who have suffered permanent, life-altering injuries.
>
> Arbitrarily limiting victims' compensation is wrong. Malpractice victims that may never be able to work again and may need help for the rest of their lives should be fairly compensated for their suffering. Without fair compensation, a terrible financial burden is imposed on their families.
>
> Those who would limit compensation for life-altering injuries say that malpractice victims still would be compensated for not being able to work, meaning, they would be compensated for their economic loss. Well, I didn't have any significant economic loss. My lost wages were approximately $8,000, and my hospital expenses of approximately $48,000 were paid for by my health insurer. My disfigurement from medical negligence is almost entirely non-economic.[9]

Yet Another View

In contrast, some other citizen groups argue that limitations on caps will help stem the tide of increasing insurance costs. Paul Becker, president of Citizens for a Sound Economy (CSE), a grassroots organization dedicated to free markets, limited government, and strong personal involvement in public policy, relays the following on the medical malpractice crisis:

> The enormous rise of premiums not only jeopardizes public health, but also increases the overall cost of healthcare in America. Doctors are being forced to use "defensive medicine" (ordering a battery of expensive tests and procedures) when they see patients, so they have a firm defense if a lawsuit is brought against them. Predictably, the costs of "defensive medicine" are passed on to consumers and taxpayers, in the form of higher healthcare premiums and taxes. In fact, a U.S. Department of Health and Human Services study found that doctors spent $6.3 billion in premiums last year and that "the direct cost of malpractice coverage and the indirect cost of defensive medicine

increases the amount the federal government must pay through these various channels, it is estimated, by $28.6 to $47.5 billion per year."[10]

H.R. 5

H.R. 5 is the Help Efficient, Accessible, Low-Cost, Timely Healthcare (HEALTH) Act of 2003. The purpose is described here:

It is the purpose of this Act to implement reasonable, comprehensive, and effective health care liability reforms designed to

1. Improve the availability of health care services in cases in which health care liability actions have been shown to be a factor in the decreased availability of services;

2. Reduce the incidence of "defensive medicine" and lower the cost of health care liability insurance, all of which contribute to the escalation of health care costs;

3. Ensure that persons with meritorious health care injury claims receive fair and adequate compensation, including reasonable non economic damages;

4. Improve the fairness and cost-effectiveness of our current health care liability system to resolve disputes over, and provide compensation for, health care liability by reducing uncertainty in the amount of compensation provided to injured individuals;

5. Provide an increased sharing of information in the health care system, which will reduce unintended injury and improve patient care.[11]

H.R. 5 was passed by the U.S. House of Representatives in March 2003. The cap was set at $250,000 for noneconomic damages of pain and suffering. The bill is currently in the Senate, and there has been a great deal of debate and disagreement over the terms and even the need for the legislation. President Bush supports its passage.

Compromises to the bill have been proposed for a "catastrophic exemption" to pain and suffering damages when an error results in significant disfigurement, disability, or death,[12] perhaps as in Linda McDougal's case. The exemption proposed would allow for awards up to $2 million. At this time, however, no comprises to the legislation have been successful.

Address the Systems

Although the debate rages on—and the crisis is a serious issue for physicians, hospitals, the insurance industry, and the legal community in the United States—malpractice litigations are not solving the predicament of medical harm. Medical malpractice still focuses on the blame factor without resolving the bigger picture of latent conditions and system failures.

Few if any settlements or jury verdicts mandate major changes in vulnerable processes that lead to system errors. Cases are solely focused on the events related to the plaintiff as economic, punitive, and other damages assessed. The broken system itself cannot be put on trial, but outcome judgments should attempt to prevent the error from recurring.

Fundamentally, findings made during the pretrial discovery period need to be explored for system commonalities that can lead to improved designs. During the pretrial period, the plaintiff's attorneys may try to use patient records or hospital information to establish a pattern of poor practice related to the claim(s) filed against the physician or hospital. Other documents related to relevance of similar nonstandard practices and trends for physicians or hospitals could demonstrate system dangers. Valuable information can be gleaned about established patterns that may lead to harm for other patients. Currently, risk management and quality departments may take data and implement changes, but there are no standardized processes to ensure this.

The High Cost of Broken Systems

In Virginia, a man entered an emergency department complaining of pain and nausea. He received Demerol for the pain and an anti-nausea drug called Phenergan. Unknown to the patient and the staff, the man was allergic to the medicines. After they were administered he went into respiratory arrest but was successfully revived. The emergency department doctor dictated the adverse event and the patient's other medical findings into the emergency department dictation system. The patient was transferred to the floor.

Several hours later, the man's pain and nausea returned. He was treated with medications. Following the injection of medicine, the man went into cardiac arrest. The code team was called. They performed CPR on him for 30 minutes and were successful in resuscitating him, but not without lacerations to his liver and spleen from the CPR. The man was hospitalized for several weeks and his medical bills totaled $75,000. The second medications that the man received were Demerol and Phenergan.

A later investigation showed that the emergency department physician had clearly dictated the adverse reaction that occurred in the emergency department; but the dictated record did not get into the patient's chart for 24 hours. All of the other communication avenues also failed. The patient sued; when the case went to trial, the jury deliberated just two-and-a-half hours. The man was awarded $305,000.[13]

Clearly, certain cases should go to trial. This man should never have received a second dose of the medicines that caused such a severe reaction. In spite of this award, no communication system overhaul was required for the hospital, and any quality improvements done by the hospital stayed within. Most settlements do not mandate system changes that would prevent other such errors.

Ask for Disclosure

Chapter 9 discussed hospital initiation of disclosure meetings. When a patient or family feels that a medical error occurred, it is appropriate for them to call the hospital executive or attorney to ask for a disclosure meeting. A consumer who conveys a desire for open, honest information exchange can help to dispel the hospital's culture of defensiveness. This is especially true if the consumer is genuinely trying to clarify facts, improve processes, and enhance patient safety.

Tips

After you have written your letters and met with hospital representatives and you are certain that an error has been committed, request a disclosure meeting with the hospital. Review the facts about the error as you know them and ask the hospital to reveal to you the findings of its investigation or root cause analysis.

When you are given your hospital admitting papers, you should also receive an information sheet outlining your patient rights and responsibilities. Carefully review this document. Provided on most rights and responsibilities disclosures are contact names, phone numbers, and addresses for the State Department of Health and the State Medical Board. Retain this information in case you need to file a complaint.

Ombudsperson (Ombudsman) Programs

Since the 1970s laws have required hospitals with subacute-care units—sometimes called transitional care units—and long-term-care facilities to display contact information about local ombudsperson organizations. Ombudsperson programs are nonprofit, independent organizations mandated by state and federal laws to protect patient rights. They are designed to assist with issues related to quality of care, financial concerns, and alleged patient abuse. Ombudspersons are trained to act as facilitators between staff and the patient or family.[14]

Mediation

Mediation is the process whereby a neutral party assists both sides of a dispute to negotiate a settlement. The mediator has no legal powers to enforce a settlement but simply works with each party, either together or independently, to reach an agreement. Generally, the costs of mediation are lower and take less time as compared to arbitration and malpractice litigation. Mediation can be a reasonable solution to disputes that are starting down the path of litigation.

The goal of mediation is to resolve differences between parties and come to agreed-upon restitution. The information discussed during mediation is confidential and cannot be used later in a lawsuit. Mediation gives the plaintiff an opportunity to air his or her perspective on the issues of restitution and to have input into determining the amount of a settlement, as opposed to a court proceeding where awards are set by a third party.[15]

Mediation can occur any time after a dispute, all the way up to a trial. It may last several hours or several days, depending on the issue. Mediators' fees start at $1,000 and range upward, depending on the attorney or legal representative.

Tip

When using a mediator, select one who has medical knowledge of your particular issue and who has superb mediation skills and experience.

At the mediation, the mediator may first meet with the attorneys and then open the general session. A summary of the issues will have been prepared by both sides' attorneys and is presented during the opening of the mediation. All parties that choose to do so can give input to their side of the issue. If a settlement is reached at the end of the mediation, then a written and binding agreement is made between the parties. If an agreement cannot be reached, then a party may proceed with further litigation.

Tips

If the first mediation was not successful, later you may elect to try mediation again, even for the same issue. You can select another mediator or mediator service. If possible, check your mediator's client references.

When undergoing mediation, ask that the hospital consider a redesign for a safer process to prevent the type of error that you experienced. You or your family may be using the services at that hospital in the future.

Arbitration

Arbitration is a process in which both parties submit a review of information to a neutral party who will make a decision that is legally binding. It differs from mediation in that a third party determines the outcome and settlement of the case instead of the two parties coming together and agreeing on the terms of the settlement. Arbitration does not always result in parties agreeing because their wishes for resolution may not have any bearing on the arbitrator's decision as he or she reviews the facts.

There are four types of arbitration: binding, nonbinding, voluntary, and mandatory. Binding arbitration means that all decisions made at the time of arbitration are final as laid out in the final written document. This form is commonly used to settle health care matters. In nonbinding arbitration, the decision can be informational and does not have to be accepted by the involved parties. Mandatory arbitration is something set in place prior to a provided service. Some doctors have patients sign agreements stating that if conflicts arise, they will be resolved through arbitration and not through litigation. Voluntary arbitration means parties agree to go to arbitration after a dispute has occurred.

Arbitration results can occur within a few days up to a few weeks. Some resolution dispute centers can assist consumers in determining the type of noncourt resolution that may be best for them.[16]

Tips

Read the paperwork in your physician's office carefully. A number of physicians, including surgeons, now ask that you sign an arbitration agreement with a refusal to sue. Arbitration may be beneficial, but just be aware that you may be signing away your right to bring a lawsuit.

Some arbitration contracts that you may sign prior to receiving care (depending on state law) allow you 30 days to reverse the agreement.

Most people don't realize they are signing an automatic arbitration agreement; they believe it is only financial paperwork.

Arbitration preparation is a crucial process. When selecting an attorney, carefully check his or her experience and expertise in medical arbitration. Thorough preparation, including discovery and joint statement of facts (facts given by both sides that are key to dispute resolution) can save significant time and cost during arbitration.

State Mandates

Several states now mandate that filed litigation malpractice cases go to a medical malpractice review panel to determine if cases can go on to arbitration or to trial. Other states mandate that medical malpractice case go directly to arbitration or mediation.

Tip

Widener University School of Law (2001) provides a Web site that describes state laws on arbitration. To review information by state on the process for arbitration and mediation laws related to medical malpractice, log on to http://www.adrlawinfo.com/medmal.html.

Settlements

Not all settlements go through the listed options. As in the case with the medical error that resulted in Ben Kolb's death, some medical errors are so serious that hospital administrators and legal teams provide an immediate financial settlement.

JASON FRANSEN

A Decision to Change

Jason Fransen, age 16, was admitted to Children's Hospital in Minneapolis with persistent pain in his right hip. After a battery of tests, he was diagnosed with a curable noncancerous disease that required eight months of treatment. Although the disease resembled cancer, it was not, and after the course of treatment, Jason was declared cured. He was given a T-shirt that said, "Jason You're Cured."

Over the next 18 months, Jason's pain returned and continued to increase. Another biopsy was performed. This test was sent out to a special children's pathologist. The results were devastating. Jason had Ewing's sarcoma, a cancerous tumor that invades the bones and certain muscle tissues. The cancer, also known as peripheral primitive neuroectodermal tumors (PNET), occurs most frequently in children between 10 and 20 and can be very vigorous. Jason went through aggressive chemotherapy, but in September 1998, the Fransens lost their son.

The Fransens filed a lawsuit against the hospital. A group of outside medical experts reviewed Jason's case. The panel found that Ewing's sarcoma was hard to diagnose. A law on the books in Minnesota said that if a patient's chance of survival was less than 40 percent at the time of diagnosis, the lawsuit could not continue. The case was dismissed.

The Fransens were devastated and extremely angry about the misdiagnosis. They asked to meet with the chief executive officer of Children's Hospital, Brock Nelson. The family wanted answers and an apology. At the meeting, although he was sympathetic, the CEO offered no further information, nor did he admit responsibility.

The meeting was a life-changing experience for Nelson. He came out of the meeting feeling horrible, saying, "It was the worst meeting I'd ever been in. We were stonewalling them."

That was the day Nelson made a decision to change the culture at Children's Hospital. He launched a patient safety revolution, starting with the practice of honest disclosure when an error occurred—who, what, where, when, and how. Safety became everyone's job, with a focus on a blame-free environment and safer system designs.

Nelson met with the Fransens, apologized, and acknowledged what happened and what steps the hospital had taken to prevent future situations like Jason's. According to the Fransens, they also received a settlement from the hospital.[17]

Dangerous Practitioners

Although their numbers are not large, there are practitioners who are incompetent, impaired, or both. Even with the safeguards of the National Practitioner Data Bank and hospital peer review systems, incompetent and impaired physicians can wreak havoc on unknowing patients.

Few regulations exist for stand-alone physician offices. A dangerous practitioner may learn to manipulate the system and avoid detection. Incompetent physicians may primarily practice outside hospitals and can go without detection for years. These doctors may avoid directly admitting patients to the hospital, and hence they shun the hospital privileging process. They may perform procedures only in their offices. These individuals must be identified and removed from practice for the protection of the public. Unless a complaint is filed with the state medical board, such practitioners may continue to practice for extended periods of time.

Tip

If you observe practices performed by a physician in the community that seem dangerous or reckless, file a complaint with the state medical board. Write down the facts in clear detail so that you can relay them accurately when you file the complaint.

Jury Trials

Jury trials are risky because no one can predict the outcome. Results vary depending on many factors, including the degree of preparation by the malpractice attorney, the strength of expert witnesses on both sides, and the perspective of any given jury. The burden of proof is on the plaintiff to show neglect or malpractice and that the care provided did not meet the acceptable standards of community practice. If the issues surrounding the error are murky, then a jury may rule in favor of the hospital or physician.

Frivolous Suits

Even though it is not a common problem, some people have learned to work the system to their advantage and look for avenues to create claims against physicians and hospitals. In Florida, Jeffery Segal, a neurosurgeon, and John R. Forbes, an attorney, have introduced a service called Medical Justice, a kind of countersuit insurance for physicians.

"Physicians who lose a lawsuit and have the insurance would be able to use a panel of lawyers gathered by U.S. Legal Services to review the case to see if it was filed frivolously or on the basis of a bad medical expert witness," Forbes explained. "If the lawyers decide that happened, the insurance company will pursue a countersuit for damages and the cost of the lawsuit. If a physician were not comfortable with the panel's decision, he or she would be able to have another person review the lawsuit."[18] Although this is a new concept, this insurance allows physicians to obtain some protection against people and attorneys who file frivolous lawsuits.

Beyond Medical Malpractice

Medical malpractice is a significant issue in the U.S. health care system, and parties on both sides of the argument feel extremely passionate. There are no easy answers to solving the issues related to perceived or real malpractice or neglect. Clearly there are times when patients and families need restitution, apologies, and closure that may be achieved through litigation. As long as health systems are in disarray, people will use litigation for resolution of errors. Perhaps through more disclosure, mediation, and meetings of hearts and minds, hospitals and patients can come to more agreements. At other times, resolution will not be possible.

Even so, partnerships between health care institutions and the public may be the beginning of change in this industry. Ideas that health care leaders cannot yet see are likely to be brought forward by the objective observers lying on the hospital beds and looking at the environment with a fresh pair of eyes. Patients often see potential changes that are not visible to physicians and other health care professionals.

Health care is on the eve of a revolution in patient safety. The joint professional-public partnership should contribute to safer system redesigns that will help to eliminate a clinician's ability to operate on the wrong side of the patient's body, run the wrong laboratory test, or administer the wrong drug. The new partnership may begin to move the public away from the need for hostile litigation that is often rightfully brought forward in today's unsafe hospital systems.

CHAPTER 11

TOWARD A NEW SAFETY CULTURE: HOW THE CHANGE WILL HAPPEN

So many of the major steps forward in our society's progress started
with just a handful of people.

—Ralph Nader, as a young Princeton student

Consumer Knowledge

Why do nurses and doctors make such bad patients? Because they
know the inherent dangers within hospitals. Most have seen serious
medical errors, and as a result, they have an overpowering need to be
in control when they receive hospital services. They are alert to the
warning signs, risks, and flaws within medical systems. They possess
one key factor that the consumer does not: knowledge. They know
how to prevent harmful events from occurring to them. Professionals
in the health care community need to view each patient as though
they or their family members were receiving medical care.

As discussed earlier, increased consumer knowledge as to the
extent of medical errors may lay the foundation for improved safety.
Equally important for patients is having the necessary confidence and
information so they can speak up and move away from assumptions.
When consumers assume too much or assume that the clinician
always knows best, so they feel they should not say anything, dangerous situations are created.

Certainly there are times when the professionals have the expertise, but clinicians are far from fail-proof. When a patient senses that he or she should speak up or identify a potential risk, that patient should do so. Accordingly, clinicians and health care workers have to refocus on the communication between themselves and the patient. Clinicians need to consistently listen to what is being said, especially if a person is voicing any type of concern—no matter the age, language, or communication barrier of the person stating the concern or question.

Partnership

The centerpiece of the patient safety transformation will be a partnership between health care professionals and the public. Consumers can help to tell hospital and organization leaders what is wrong and what they want to see changed.

Limited pressure is being placed on state and federal legislative bodies, and a few safety organizations are starting to improve available information on patient safety (see "Patient Safety Resources" in appendix 2). Despite this, the public is still deficient in knowledge of the specific risks of potential medical errors, and it lacks the means and empowerment to organize efforts to make real change to reduce medical errors.

Listen to Those Who May Have an Idea

In the 1950s, a young Princeton University student walking to class early one morning noticed some dead robins and bluebirds by a big tree. As he looked around, he noticed more dead birds. In the following days, the student watched the groundskeepers spraying the trees around the campus with big hoses emitting a whitish substance. Each morning, the groundskeepers would pick up the dead birds and dispose of them.

The young student decided to go to the student newspaper, the *Daily Princetonian*. He asked the editors to do an article on the situation. He took one of the dead birds with him to show the editors what was happening. The editors said, "There's nothing wrong. We have some of the best science professors in the world, chemistry, biology. If they had any idea that it was harmful, it would be stopped." Nothing was written in the student newspaper, and the spraying continued for years.

The substance that was being sprayed was DDT, the deadly pesticide that was strictly banned in the 1970s.[1] The student was Ralph Nader.

Tips

When you are hospitalized, the care you receive may progress rapidly. New medication and treatment options will be ordered depending on your illness or injury. Continue to seek information on each new course of treatment. Ask your physician to provide additional consultations on new treatments and medications. Depending on the treatment, you can consult with other physicians, specialized nurses, dietitians, social workers, therapists, and chaplains. In nonemergency situations, if you are uncertain about something, do not feel pressured to make decisions until you have the facts you need. Ask your nurse to explain information on the medications you are receiving, including IV medications.

When you or your family member are being admitted to the hospital under urgent or emergency circumstances, you can delay signing financial, patient rights, or the Health Insurance Portability and Accountability Act (HIPAA) paperwork. Once you are sure that you or your family member are taken care of, then you can sit down and read all the paperwork. You can also ask for help and review the paperwork with a hospital representative.

History of Other Consumer Change

Consumers should begin to pressure the health care industry and legislative bodies to deploy more rapid implementation of a patient safety culture. The current change is slow, as evidenced by system failures that recently resulted in the deaths of Jesica Santillán and Gianni Vargas. Both deaths occurred long after the Institute of Medicine's report was released.

In 1995, the CEO of Delta Airlines stated, "Safety is Delta's top priority every hour of every day." And a CEO of a major automobile manufacturer announced, "Safety is a customer's right." The health care industry and its leaders can ask no less than this. Even so, these statements and slogans did not come about without pressure from consumers, pilots, drivers, and passengers who demanded improvements in air and road safety.

As early as the 1950s, the air force found it was losing more of its personnel to accidents than it was losing in the Korean War. It did not take long for the leaders of aviation to begin to make improvement in air safety.

In the 1960s, many traffic accidents that resulted in devastating harm such as brain injuries, massive abdominal injuries, and death were blamed solely on the driver. Certainly driver error and human factors did contribute to accidents, and continue to do so today, but at that time the cars were just plain unsafe. Broken windshield glass would shatter like ice, lap belts were worthless in preventing head trauma, steering columns would end up on the ceiling, doors would fling open during the collision, children were improperly restrained (if they were restrained at all), seats would collapse, engines and dashboards would end up on top of the driver, and other design flaws also contributed to death and harm. These defective designs were not the fault of the driver.

In the 1960s, things began to change. The public learned about "Sierra Sam" ("born" in 1949), the first crash-test dummy.

When crash-test dummies were introduced, there was an awakening to what actually happened during an automobile collision. Films displayed cars folding up like accordions and the crash-test dummies crumpling like paper. As they watched, consumers thought, "That could be me, or my children." They began to realize that automobile design factors were contributing to injuries and death, and they started to focus attention on the problem of flawed design in automobiles. The next step was to pressure the U.S. Congress to enact legislation for the design of safer vehicles. Because of this, over time, the automobile industry had to design solutions to prevent the vehicle accordion phenomenon.

Initially, the automobile industry resisted change amid concerns that expensive designs would jack up prices and cause automakers to lose their market. They were suspicious and mistrustful of consumer advocates and grassroots organizations for automobile safety. Motives and agendas were questioned, and private investigators were hired to tail critics of unsafe automobile designs and look into their private affairs.

Consumer knowledge began to increase. It took consumer pressure and legislative action by Congress to promote changes. Through diligent work on the part of the advocate leaders, members of Congress began to learn about the dangers of automobile accidents. Congress was influenced to legislate improvements in auto safety design that would prevent injuries and fatalities. Unfortunately, it also took stories and testimonies of personal tragedies caused by poorly designed vehicles to have an impact, all of which helped to accelerate the changes in the U.S. automobile industry.

In 1966, Congress passed the Motor Vehicle Safety Act. The act launched the beginning of other legislation focused on traffic safety.

In 1970, the Highway Safety Act was established, which led to the founding of the National Highway Traffic Safety Administration (NHTSA) under the Department of Transportation.

> NHTSA is responsible for reducing deaths, injuries and economic losses resulting from motor vehicle crashes. NHTSA express duties are listed in the following:
>
> > Investigates safety defects in motor vehicles, sets and enforces fuel economy standards, helps states and local communities reduce the threat of drunk drivers, promotes the use of safety belts, child safety seats and air bags, investigates odometer fraud, establishes and enforces vehicle anti-theft regulations and provides consumer information on motor vehicle safety topics.
>
> NHTSA conducts research on driver behavior and traffic safety and to develop the most efficient and effective means of bringing about safety improvements.[2]

Parallels between Patient and Automotive Safety

Some stark differences exist between the current dilemma of medical errors and past issues in automobile safety. Since the Institute of Medicine's report was released in 1999, health care leaders and organizations such as the JCAHO have embraced the fact that there is a peril of medical harm and adverse events affecting patients today. In contrast to the automobile industry of the 1960s, which resisted costly overhauls in automotive safety, there is little resistance from the health care community about the dangers within hospitals. Results of the IOM report and numerous other studies continue to show the prevalence of medical errors. However, the means to overhaul patient safety are yet to be established.

Many comparisons have been made between safety advancements in the automotive industry and those in patient safety. Looking at these comparisons helps to crystallize where pressure is needed in order to effect change in the health care industry.

Automotive Safety *(1960–current)*	*Patient Safety* *(1999–current)*
1. Denial by the industry of the extent of the problem	1. Recognition by the industry of the extent of the problem
2. Effective lobbying pressure	2. Minimal lobbying pressure
3. Extensive public pressure	3. Increasing public pressure

4. Legislative change	4. Beginning of legislative change
5. Competition of foreign markets with extensive automobile safety features (e.g., Volvo, Mercedes)	5. No direct competition exists; however, a factor exists that if the private industry is unable to solve the problem of medical errors, then government-run or nationalized health care is possible. Many Americans strongly resist this concept.
6. Research	6. Research
7. Automotive profits to design safer domestic automobiles	7. Minimal funding for safety redesign
8. Automotive safety changes	8. Slow patient safety changes

Clearly, patient safety is still in its infancy. Nonetheless, lobbying and public pressure must be increased, as well as legislative change. The lack of competition and market profits have to be recognized and feasible planning and solutions employed. Then, perhaps, the health care industry will not have to wait several decades to drive improvements in health care.

To show that health care professionals recognize dangerous systems, surveys of health care professionals continue to support the high numbers of medical errors witnessed by physicians, nurses, and other clinicians. Given these findings, there is little doubt that patient harm is a serious issue. This acknowledgement gives the health care industry an advantage over the automobile industry in its willingness to admit that a problem exists. Fear of losing the market because of the costs involved in implementing safety features is not the key issue of slow change in patient safety improvement. As we have seen over and over again in the cases discussed throughout this book, errors, inefficiencies, handoffs, and duplications that set the stage for errors appear to be more costly in terms of human resources, dollar expenditures, and patient harm than the redesign of safer systems. Health care leaders and practitioners possess the motivation to make these changes; the means to change, however, are challenging.

Although the publicity surrounding the IOM report has helped make the public more knowledgeable about some risks of medical errors, consumers are still not continually informed about the full scope of the problem. They also are not fully aware of how they can directly influence the health care industry. This change will take place more readily with additional consumer-focused research, educational material about error factors, and accessible resources on error prevention. In addition, strong consumer organizations that proactively influence and lobby for improvements in patient safety are greatly needed.

After the release of "To Err Is Human," the general media focused on stories of medical harm and the report's shocking conclusions; more recently, however, little focus from the media is given to the subject of medical errors, other than an occasional story. Until the layers of harm are peeled back, little will be revealed about this dilemma. A few professional patient safety organizations have been influential with some proposed legislation; yet on the whole, consumer groups need to place much more pressure on state and federal legislative bodies and work toward error prevention. When an incident such as the one that involved Jesica Santillán occurs, there is a tremendous focus of concern on medical errors, yet consistent efforts seem to stop when the media flurry dies down. Permanent changes in hospital system design will occur with mandated safety technologies and appropriate ongoing data. (More will be discussed on data in chapter 12.)

Tools of Change

Fully Integrated Electronic Medical Records

According to the IOM, a functional electronic medical record (EMR) has the following components:

1. Health information and data: Immediate access to key information that would improve the ability of clinicians to make sound decisions in a timely manner. Those data include patients' diagnoses, allergies, and laboratory test results.

2. Results management: Quick access of new and past test results by all clinicians involved in treating a patient.

3. Order management: Computerized entry and storage of data on all medications, tests, and other services.

4. Decision support: Electronic alerts and reminders to improve compliance with best practices, ensure regular screenings and other preventive practices, identify possible drug interactions, and facilitate diagnoses and treatments.

5. Electronic communication and connectivity: Secure and readily accessible communication among clinicians and patients.

6. Patient support: Tools offering patients access to their medical records, interactive education, and the ability to do home monitoring and self-testing.

7. Administrative processes: Tools, including scheduling systems that improve administrative efficiencies and patient service.

8. Reporting: Electronic data storage that uses uniform data standards to enable physician offices and health care organizations to comply with federal, state, and private reporting requirements in a timely manner.[3]

Currently, a number of hospitals and health care systems are designing and implementing computerized physician order entry (CPOE) systems as discussed earlier. However, use of entirely integrated EMR systems is limited because the cost of implementation is enormous, ranging from $1 million in small facilities to greater than $40 million in large, integrated hospital systems. Exact cost figures will become clear in retrospect as more hospitals implement EMR. The products are expensive, and so is the labor required to study, evaluate, select, and start up an EMR. Cost factors affect clinics, outpatient settings, and doctors' offices as well.

Earlier in the book, the fragmentation of hospital computer systems was discussed. In this chapter we review the challenges of integrating mixed manual and electronic documentation systems. As components of computer systems have infiltrated the health care market, most hospitals have portions of patient records on "niche" (stand-alone) computer systems.

The array of mixed manual and electronic information sources include items such as electronic nurses' charting, but handwritten physician orders; dictated notes on operations, but handwritten anesthesia records; computerized laboratory systems, but handwritten progress notes. (Progress notes are a crucial document physicians use to track the daily progress of patients. Medical errors have occurred because of documentation issues on these handwritten notes.)

The challenge for hospitals—given their limited financial resources—is how to move toward an entire computerized patient medical record that is affordable, integrated, and safe. The task is tremendous, and there is hardly a hospital in the United States that is not grappling with this issue. The easiest solution is to simply replace all niche products with one fully integrated electronic system. Unfortunately, this is not an option for most hospitals because of financial limitations for such sweeping purchases and integration of the applications.

Hence, hospitals are faced with decisions regarding stair-step upgrades, such as implementing a CPOE but delaying an entire EMR or placing an EMR only in the outpatient area, and safely interfacing niche systems. Given the economics of the health care industry, hospitals that are making upgrades to an integrated EMR are taking great financial risks. Boards and hospital executives are weighing the risks of integrating EMRs while recognizing that the current patient systems are increasingly inadequate to meet the advancing needs of medicine.

Numerous prospective financial analyses (usually performed by individual hospitals) and a few retrospective studies have been performed to evaluate the return on investment of an EMR, but at this time in health care, there is little hard, long-standing data to say from a purely financial standpoint that an electronic medical record will have significant positive financial returns. Therefore, many leaders are making the decision to move forward with an EMR to improve patient safety and to stay current with today's technology demands.

The Medication Errors Reduction Act

Senators Bob Graham (D-FL) and Olympia Snowe (R-ME) have proposed legislation to provide funding for hospitals and skilled nursing facilities to integrate information technologies that improve patient safety. The Medication Errors Reduction Act proposes $97.5 million per year for the installation of CPOEs, EMRs, and electronic dispensing technologies. The grants would be available until 2011 to help offset the costs of error-reducing technology. Currently, the Senate is reviewing the bill. Although this act may provide some financial assistance, given the numbers of hospitals and long-term-care facilities in the United States, the legislation does not address the cost issues as a whole. More information is provided in chapter 12, under "Patient Safety and Public Health Legislation."

Tips

Computerized entry systems are susceptible to data entry errors. Always ask for a printout of your paperwork and review the information for accuracy.

Each time you receive hospital or health care services, check the information in your patient documents to make sure it is still correct. Especially important is your medication history and allergy status.

If your health or medication status has changed, update the information immediately and watch to assure the entry is made in the computer. Then recheck a printed copy of your information for accuracy.

Resistance to Change

In theory, physicians and health care professionals recognize that a computerized patient record is important; nevertheless, initiating a new system can be an overwhelming change for an institution. Patient data are the foundation of a hospital's daily work; when this is overhauled, it can create havoc and even fear among professionals. There have been physician revolts when, instead of being voluntary, allowing a choice between the old manual charting and the new electronic charting, CPOE products have been mandated. The process of how to implement an EMR—including physician buy-in—is as vital for hospitals as which EMR product to select. Because this is a new and massive change, little experience exists as to the best way(s) for physicians and professionals to accept and utilize EMRs.

Better Information for Physicians

"Medical ignorance is widely assumed to be the cause of errors in medical practice," wrote Clement J. McDonald, M.D., in a 1976 article appearing in the *New England Journal of Medicine*. In an era of heightened awareness of the pervasiveness of medical errors in this country's health care system, for many that statement still rings true today. However, a quarter century ago Dr. McDonald set out to prove his hypothesis that *many medical errors are due to the physician's intrinsic limits rather than to remedial flaws in his fund of knowledge.*

McDonald is now the director of the Regenstrief Institute and a professor of medicine at Indiana University School of Medicine. He writes, "The computer augments the physician's capabilities and thereby reduces his error rate."[4]

An EMR has the potential to enhance how and what a physician receives as valuable clinical data. Because the majority of decisions physicians make are based on data—the patient's symptoms, blood test results, imaging studies, blood pressure and heart rate—the volume of data reviewed each day by a given physician is significant. Faster and more accurate transmission of information may reduce potential errors. Still, some doctors resist the change because they perceive the old manual systems as reliable and believe they function adequately with them.

Among physicians, there are early adapters who embrace the new technology and take full advantage of the electronic systems. Although the age of the physician can be a factor, resistance to change is not necessarily related to age. Some older doctors have led the drive to install computerized systems, and some younger physicians have fiercely opposed the change.

Brigham and Women's Hospital

The Brigham and Women's Hospital in Boston has put an EMR system into operation. Its system incorporates many of the components listed in the IOM report, including CPOE, clinical decision support, and cost-accounting functions. Brigham and Women's Hospital has over 5,600 computer workstations.

Jeffery Otten, president and CEO of Brigham and Women's Hospital, stated:

> The results of error reduction, improvements in patient safety and financial saving for Brigham and Women's Hospital have been significant. The return on investment, in terms of both enhancing patient safety and improving the hospital's bottom line, is staggering. The BIC system has reduced medical errors at Brigham and Women's by 55 percent, saving the hospital between $5 million and $10 million a year. Patient allergy warnings result in 60 percent to 70 percent of orders being cancelled. Drug interaction warnings result in a 100 percent change in orders. 50 percent of orders are changed when the system indicates that an order or test has already been administered.[5]

It Takes Time

The money and the complexities involved in implementing EMR systems are enormous; in addition, the time it takes to install an electronic system is just as much of a limitation to hospitals as the dollars. The time required to install a CPOE system, in general, is significantly underestimated at the onset of most projects. The delays are multiple. Resources can be limited because people, technology, and other urgent health care issues frequently arise. The onset of bioterrorism threats, anthrax scares, smallpox worries, illnesses such as severe acute respiratory syndrome (SARS) and West Nile virus, and newly enacted regulations may shift dollars and resources to other important immediate needs.

According to Suzanne Delbanco, executive director of the Leapfrog Group, "[Currently], only 2.5 percent of hospitals have fully implemented computerized drug ordering systems."[6] More recently, up to 5 percent of the hospitals participating in the Leapfrog Group report that they have a CPOE. Keep in mind that this number represents hospitals that have responded to the Leapfrog survey; it does not represent all U.S. hospitals. Although it is not known for sure, hospitals participating in Leapfrog may be more aggressive in implementing safety technology.

JIM

A Model of What the Consumer Is Coming to Expect

Jim, age 49, has recently been diagnosed with diabetes. Although his father died of complications from diabetes and heart disease, Jim is determined to beat the odds. He sits down at his computer to peruse the Internet and finds out about preventing diabetes complications. He logs on to the American Diabetes Association Web site and reads about foot care as well as kidney and heart disease prevention. Jim is 30 pounds overweight and suffers from high blood pressure.

As he searches the Internet, Jim reads about a drug known as an ACE (angiotensin converting enzyme) inhibitor. He reads how the drug can help prevent kidney disease in people with diabetes and high blood pressure. He sends an e-mail off to his doctor inquiring whether this medication would be helpful for him. Jim orders his diabetes medication from an online pharmacy and receives monthly electronic reminders when it is time to reorder.

When Jim was first diagnosed with diabetes, he saw a dietitian who gave him some Internet resources. He was able to download sample menus for his diabetes diet.

As Jim is reading about appropriate exercise options for people with diabetes, he receives an e-mail reply from his primary doctor telling him that at his next appointment, the doctor will evaluate Jim for a medication called Monopril, which is an ACE inhibitor. His doctor agrees with Jim that this could help him prevent kidney disease and help control Jim's high blood pressure.

Jim monitors his blood sugar and downloads the previous week's results from his glucose monitor to the computer. The results are graphed out and he e-mails them to his endocrinologist, who will be seeing him later that week. She will have several days to evaluate Jim's blood sugar control and prepare recommendations before he arrives for his appointment.

Health consumers are coming to expect these conveniences and enhancements when receiving health care services. The rapid growth of computer technology and the Internet provides the public with more health care information than has been available at any other time in history.

Consumers as Recipients

Hospital leaders and information technology departments are working hard on the rollout of CPOEs and EMRs. However, few if any of these teams involve consumers. It might benefit the health care community to solicit input from former patients so that the recipient's perception of the products is incorporated into the technology design. As end users of services, the patients can identify both the positive and negative aspects of these products.

One of the cultural norms within hospitals is that clinician input is central to new changes, but hospital leaders miss valuable input from the patients. Using consumer focus groups to solicit ideas and perspectives on what did and did not work with current electronic systems might provide valuable insights during the implementation of EMR pilot programs.

Tips

Ask your hospital or health care system if it uses consumer focus groups for safety. If it does, consider participating in the groups. Often the hospital may provide small incentives such as gift certificates to the participants.

If you receive a hospital survey, complete it. Add handwritten comments if the survey does not address your concerns. Hospitals do evaluate and make changes in response to patient survey results.

Using human factors engineering such as occurred in the early development of aviation and the nuclear power industry may help to offset design flaws in hospital technology systems. Most likely, EMRs will significantly enhance patient safety; nevertheless, the new systems are still tools and as such are subject to other types of unforeseen errors. Proactively using consumer input and human factors engineering during the design phase may assist in foreseeing latent conditions that could be built into new electronic products.

Bar Coding

Bar coding identification is a technology that supermarkets have used consistently for well over two decades. The use of bar coding is so common that the consumer hardly is aware of the practice, that is, until a buyer selects an item that is not bar coded. Shoppers in the checkout line wait anxiously while a store employee gets a manual price check. At that moment, consumers have a great appreciation for bar-coded products.

FDA Mandates Bar Coding in Medications in Hospitals

In February 2004 the FDA published a ruling to mandate bar coding of medications dispensed to hospitalized patients. The FDA projects that this practice has the potential to decrease adverse events by 500,000 and to save $93 billion over the next two decades. These savings are expected to come from decreased harm to patients, fewer days spent by patients in the hospital, less litigation, and more effective billing of medications. A fully implemented bar coding system works in conjunction with an EMR as follows:

1. A bar-coded identification bracelet or tag is given to the patient upon admission to the hospital.
2. The bar code contains the patient's medical information and is linked to the patient's EMR. The EMR includes a bar coding scanner.
3. The hospital medications are premarked with a bar code, which is called a national drug code (NDC) identifier.
4. The nurse or clinician pulls up the patient's information in the computer and scans the medication's NDC.
5. The patient's information is electronically matched with the drug NDC to ensure it is the appropriate medication for that patient, including correct drug, dose, time to be given, and administration method.
6. If any information is incorrect, an error message is electronically generated, warning the nurse or clinician of the problem. This allows him or her to make the needed corrections before any drug is administered.[7]

Pharmaceutical manufacturers will have two years to place NDC codes on current medications. Medications newly approved by the FDA will require NDC codes. The consumer must keep in mind that bar coding technology will be dependent on the implementation of EMR and bar coding systems within hospitals. As of March 2004, according to the American Medical Association, fewer than 2 percent of hospitals have bar coding systems.[8]

Bar coding technology within hospitals can be used for multiple other purposes such as coding laboratory tests, surgical procedure identification, radiology tests, and keeping better track of patient product charges. Today, product charge coding is the most frequently used type of bar coding in hospitals. This was driven largely by the product manufacturers, who began bar coding when the technology was introduced.

SANG

Sang had a family history of colon cancer. His mother died of the disease when she was 42. Sang, now 37, was told by his physician that he should have a colonoscopy to assess his risk for cancer. So Sang was scheduled for the procedure.

The morning of the procedure, the admissions clerk registered Sang in the computer. He was given a wristband with a bar code. Sang's doctor had ordered some laboratory blood work to evaluate his general health history, so Sang first went to the hospital lab. His laboratory order had a bar code on it, and both Sang and the order were scanned. Everything matched up correctly. After the blood work, Sang proceeded to the outpatient procedure suite.

Sang was instructed as to what would happen during the colonoscopy. He was brought to the procedure room and an IV was started. As the nurse prepared the medications for Sang's sedation, she scanned the medicines in the syringes and then scanned Sang's wristband. The first two medications scanned fine. When the nurse scanned the third medication, a warning came up on the computer and stopped her from proceeding further: "Patient Allergic to Darvacet, DO NOT ADMINISTER DEMEROL." When Sang had registered, he had told the admitting clerk that he was allergic to Darvacet, a mild narcotic. The computer and the bar coding automatically recorded that all related narcotics were contraindicated for Sang, hence stopping a direct IV injection of Demerol, a potent narcotic. The Demerol was sent back to the pharmacy and replaced with another medication that was nonnarcotic.

Tip

Be alert if you have a common last name such as Garcia, Smith, or Jones, and especially so if you also have a common first name like Jose, Mary, or Bob. Name confusion is a common problem that can lead to errors. The hospital unit will generally put a name alert reminder on patient information when there are two patients with the same name. This reminder does not guarantee an error-free process, however. You must be extra diligent to ensure that all tests, medications, information exchanges, or procedures are intended for you.

Telecommunication and Fiscal Limitations

The prevalence of telecommunication and electronic technology in the form of cell phones, Internet links, voice recognition dictation, wireless servers, and handheld computers is increasing in hospitals. Many physicians now contain patient information in Palm Pilot computers. Some personal digital assistant (PDA) systems available for nursing units allow nurses to chart and track patient information at the bedside, eliminating reliance on paper and the need to chart manually at a later time.

Budget constraints continue to be problematic for hospitals and hinder quicker implementation of electronic systems. Every new proposed electronic product has to be weighed carefully for how it can be integrated with other electronic systems.

Private grants for implementing electronic systems are scarce and come with limitations. Fund-raising is helpful, but it has its limitations, too. Donors may be excited about giving money for a new pediatrics wing, but donating for a new computer system just does not produce the same interest.

Personal Electronic Medical Record

In April 2004, President George W. Bush set a goal for most Americans to have an electronic medical record within the next 10 years. In a speech at the Baltimore Veterans Affairs Medical Center, Bush stated that medical records are "still in the buggy era." This proposal calls for a nationwide computerized patient record that links hospital, pharmacy, and other medical information. Also, an overview of the White House proposal mentions electronic prescribing as a way to reduce medication errors. Bush's 2005 budget proposes $100 million for government-funded information technologies. The president also proposed the creation of a national information technology coordinator to oversee the project.[9]

Health Care at a Crossroads

Health care is at a crossroads. Improvements in patient safety are paramount. Although not every medical error can be prevented, according to the IOM, at least 50 percent of the adverse events that occur in health care may be decreased with creative preventive steps.

As with automobiles, hospital environments and health care systems have to be made "crash-worthy" for patients. Perhaps the medical community would benefit from a type of "hospital crash-test dummy" to test out new systems and technologies and drive home the importance of error-proofing enhancements. Since automotive safety strategies were implemented, not all road fatalities have been stopped. Automobiles were improved, but not before consumers realized that the cars of the 1950s and 1960s killed many more people than they had to. The driver of any vehicle still has to be responsible, as does each health care provider, but a number of immediate technologies and safety changes can be implemented to begin the "crashworthiness" of hospitals.

CHAPTER 12

THE PATIENT PARTNERSHIP: WHAT NEEDS TO CHANGE

New Rules

As a follow-up to its 1999 report "To Err Is Human," the Institute of Medicine released another report in 2001 called "Crossing the Quality Chasm: A New Health System for the 21st Century."[1] This report focused on six aims that should be central when receiving medical services: safety, effectiveness, patient-centeredness, timeliness, efficiency, and equity. The report stated that the aims should be complementary and synergistic and that in the current systems these aims are visibly missing. The report noted, "The health care system currently does not, as a whole, make the best use of its resources."

The IOM report revealed that achieving these aims will require a new and profound change. An entirely redesigned framework is needed. The IOM focused on 10 new rules for rebuilding the United States' health system, which should move health care into an era of enhanced patient knowledge and open communication between patients and providers.

In addition to the new rules that the IOM is recommending, an even stronger focus on partnerships is required. Beyond a set of principles, there must be a shift in the daily functioning between patients and providers. The clinician–customer relationship must be enhanced with respect and service-minded thinking. Patients can no longer feel as if they are "in the way." This sets the stage for errors.

Table 12.1
Patient Partnership Principles

Current Approach (IOM)	New Rule (IOM 2001)	Patient Partnership Principles
Care is based primarily on visits.	1. Care is based on a continuous healing relationship.	1. The patient is the center of the continuous healing relationship.
Professional autonomy (independence) drives variability.	2. Care is customized according to the patient s needs and values.	2. Remove barriers and obstacles to learning about the patient s needs and values.
Professional controlled care.	3. The patient is the source of control.	3. Ask the patients how obstacles can be eliminated and how the patient can gain more control of their health care. Move beyond patient satisfaction surveys.
Information is a record.	4. Knowledge is shared and information flows freely.	4. Provide all information to patients about the course of treatment at the onset of a course of treatment. Remove the piecemeal dispersion of information that hinder patient planning and knowledge.
Decision making is based on training and experience.	5. Decision making is based on evidence.	5. Present all evidenced-based options to the patient at the start of treatment.
Do no harm is an individual responsibility.	6. Safety is a system property.	6. Safety is a shared partnership with the health care consumer.
Secrecy is necessary.	7. Transparency is necessary.	7. See the patient at the center of the transparency.
The system reacts to needs.	8. Needs are anticipated.	8. Ask the patient what his or her needs are.
Cost reduction is sought.	9. Waste is continuously decreased.	9. Don t create more redundancies and duplications for the health care consumer.
Preference is given to professional roles over the system.	10. Cooperation among clinicians is a priority.	10. Cooperation between clinicians and patients is paramount.

Source: Simple Rules for Twenty-First-Century Health Care System—New Patient Partnership Principles (Institute of Medicine).

Just for a moment, imagine arriving at an electronics store with cash in hand to purchase a television, and being ignored, then belittled, and rudely addressed by the clerk on the floor. Your order is lost and the wrong product arrives. Most consumers would choose to go to a different store. In health care a perception has developed in which substandard service and inefficiency are tolerated since consumers are not usually paying directly for care, even though they regularly make co-payments. Perhaps if co-payments were $100 instead of $10 people would expect greater service and more efficiency.

Yet, as outlined in many studies, Americans are paying for these inefficiencies through increasing insurance premiums, higher co-payments, and higher product and service costs that are passed on by businesses to cover their health care costs. Fragmented services also cause waste and increased opportunity for error. Patients feel less knowledgeable than their health care workers and may elect not to speak up when they feel they are in the way, even when they sense something is out of place. This is especially true when a patient enters a hospital. Certainly consumers cannot know all the nuances of hospital service, but they should have an increased knowledge base and not be intimidated when speaking up. Patients should expect increased efficiencies from both a safety and a service perspective. Yet health care consumers need tools and data to accomplish this. Provided here are the recommended aims and additional principles, along with a case study, that are needed to begin the shift in the patient–provider relationship.

The New Rules Are Not in Place

The new IOM rules are not yet in place, nor have reasonable partnerships been formed with patients. This is evidenced not only by errors but also by the overuse and waste that plays out every day in U.S. hospitals and health care arenas, as displayed in the continuing scenario with Mrs. U (see chapter 2).

More on Mrs. U

Mrs. U went for her second visit to the orthopedic surgeon after her MRI was completed. The MRI showed significantly more damage to her right shoulder than the X-ray. In addition to the cyst, Mrs. U had a rotator cuff tear and needed surgery. Mrs. U was told that she would need an electrocardiogram (ECG) before the procedure but that her primary doctor would have to do this. The results of the MRI had been with the surgeon for over a week, and the staff knew that surgery would be indicated.

Mrs. U had just seen her primary doctor the day before her appointment with her surgeon. However, Mrs. U. had another routine appointment with her diabetes doctor scheduled for the next day. Because of this, the orthopedic surgeon told Mrs. U she could have her diabetes doctor do the 12-lead ECG, hence avoiding another appointment with the primary doctor.

> *Patient Partnership Principle: 4. Provide all information about the course of treatment to the patient at the onset of a diagnosis. Remove the "piecemeal" dispersion of information that hinders patient knowledge and planning.*

The following day, when Mrs. U arrived for her appointment with her diabetes doctor, she told her doctor what the surgeon had said about the ECG. Her doctor said, "Yes, we can do the ECG." After the doctor went to see the next patient, the nurse told Mrs. U that she would not do the ECG because the insurance did not allow it.

> *Patient Partnership Principles: 1. The patient is at the center of the healing relationship. 7. See the patient at the center of the transparency.*

The nurse said that the diabetes doctor was not the primary doctor and that Mrs. U would have to see her primary doctor for the ECG.

> *Patient Partnership Principles: 2. Remove barriers and obstacles to learning about the patient's needs and values. 9. Don't create more redundancies and duplications for the health care consumer.*

Mrs. U explained to the nurse that she would now have to go back to her primary doctor's office, where she had just been, and that she was not seeing that doctor again before surgery. Mrs. U asked, "Could you please do the ECG?" The diabetes doctor's nurse refused, saying it had to be done by the primary doctor.

> *Patient Partnership Principle: 8. Ask the patient what his or her needs are.*

Mrs. U offered to pay cash for the ECG. She did not want to schedule yet another doctor's visit, and her primary doctor was a one-hour trip from her home. In addition, another doctor's appointment would significantly impact Mrs. U's work schedule. Meanwhile, the ECG machine was sitting in the hallway while the discussion took place. The nurse again refused to do the ECG, saying, "It's against the rules."

> *Patient Partnership Principle: 10. Cooperation between clinicians and patients is paramount.*

While the discussion about the ECG was going on between Mrs. U and the nurse, Mrs. U received a call on her cell phone from her orthopedic surgeon's office, saying they now needed to schedule a history and physical appointment with the orthopedic surgeon before the surgery.

> *Patient Partnership Principle: 3. Ask the patient how obstacles can be eliminated and how the patient can gain more control over his or her health care. Move beyond patient satisfaction surveys.*

Instances similar to Mrs. U's fragmented care occur regularly in health care. Her case is also a key example of how her ECG could have been missed between all of her doctors. Because Mrs. U had had diabetes for 34 years and also had high blood pressure and kidney disease, she was at a high risk for cardiac complications during surgery. If Mrs. U had not been educated about her health issues, she might have given up in frustration and not have had a presurgical ECG.

Patient Partnership Principle: 6. Safety is a shared partnership with the health care consumer.

If the ECG was not done and a cardiac complication occurred during surgery that could have been prevented, then the adverse event might just be chalked up to "the patient's condition." The surgeon might have noticed the missing ECG, if he remembered, or it may have been excluded because of the fragmentation. Also, the extra cost has to be considered, given that Mrs. U's insurance was paying for each additional visit; these multiple visits could have been streamlined if the care had been coordinated.

The Cost of U.S. Health Care

U.S. health care is one of the most costly medical care systems in the world. Expenditures for medical care in the United States have been calculated at $1 trillion per year, which accounts for 15 percent of the gross national product.

As referenced earlier, the Midwest Business Group on Health's 2003 report stated that "30% of all direct health care outlays today are the result of poor quality health care consisting primarily of overuse, misuse and waste."[2] The treatment of Mrs. U is just one simple example of inefficiency and waste. As these cases are duplicated every hour, every day in U.S. health care systems, the 30 percent of waste is easy to spot. This type of expense, with its inefficiencies, dangers, and waste, would not be tolerated in any other U.S. trade. If health care were any other private enterprise, it likely would be out of business. Other kinds of commerce simply would not survive. Certainly, improvements in decreasing waste, duplications, inefficiencies, and misuse need to occur rapidly. The frustration, extra time, and extra energy spent by health care consumers also have to be considered as motivations for decreasing this waste.

Tips

Once you are told you need surgery, start a notepad.

In your notepad, write down all of the questions you want to ask your surgeon.

Initially, talk to your surgeon and review and document in your notepad all the things your surgeon wants you to do before the procedure.

When you are first told that you need surgery, ask immediately what other tests and preparations you will need before the surgery. Ask who will be performing the tests and when they need to be done. Write all this information in your notepad.

Check off each test and preparation as it is completed. Note the date of each procedure, who performed it, and the place it was performed.

At least two days before the scheduled surgery, check with your surgeon's office to ensure that he or she has received all the results of your completed tests and preparations.

Confirm with the surgeon's office that on the day of your surgery, all of your test results and paperwork will be available at the hospital or outpatient surgery center.

In your notepad, write down the medications you will be receiving, including the antibiotic type and the time you are to receive it before your incision. Check the names of the medications for accurate spelling and confirm the names with your surgeon.

Speak on the phone or schedule an appointment with your anesthesiologist before surgery. Review with the anesthesiologist the antibiotic and timing that your surgeon reviewed with you. See the anesthesiology tips in chapter 7.

For many surgeries, including bone, cardiac, and abdominal surgeries, showering before surgery is a step that can help prevent infection. Depending on the type of surgery, the Centers for Disease Control recommend specific guidelines for presurgery showering (such as with a special soap that your doctor can recommend; many of these are over-the-counter solutions). Discuss with your surgeon his or her showering recommendations for the type of surgery that you are having.

At least 10 days before surgery, review all your medicines with your surgeon. Include prescription medications, supplements, vitamins, minerals, and herbs. Determine whether any medicines you are taking contain hidden aspirin products. Discuss your aspirin product use with your surgeon. He or she may want you to discontinue aspirin products 10 days before surgery, but be sure to ask your doctor's advice; do not decide on your own.

Advisory Council for Health Care

Two newly formed organizations now focus on improved quality and safety in health care. Kenneth Kizer, one of the authors of "To Err Is Human," spoke about the need for two new organizations to help improve safety and quality in U.S. health systems. The first, a private, nonprofit membership organization called the National Forum on Health Care Quality Measurement and Reporting—primarily consisting of health care professionals—was originally proposed by the President's Advisory Commission on Consumer Protection and Quality in the Health Care Industry. And the second, the Advisory Council for Health Care, would focus more on health care consumers:

> The concept of the National Quality Forum arose in recognition of a strong American sentiment against government regulation and control of healthcare quality. Of note, the Commission proposed a public-private partnership involving two new organizations.
>
> Those organizations included a private-sector entity they referred to as the National Forum on Health Care Quality Measurement and Reporting (better known now as the National Quality Forum, or NQF) and a public entity they called the Advisory Council for Health Care Quality. The Commission's original vision was that the Advisory Council would identify national goals for quality improvement and provide oversight on the accomplishment of those goals, while the NQF would devise a national strategy for measuring and reporting healthcare quality that would advance the identified national aims for improvement.
>
> The NQF believes that it must always ensure that the consumer perspective is heard during the discussion of quality measures. In an effort to continuously actualize this, the NQF Board of Directors is designed to have a majority of its members representing consumers and purchasers. This is an important structural precept that should facilitate keeping the consumer perspective ever present.[3]

National Mandated Reporting System

Recommendation 5.1 in "To Err Is Human" states:

> A nationwide mandatory reporting system should be established that provides for the collection of standardized information by state governments about adverse events that result in death or serious harm. Reporting should initially be required by hospitals and eventually be required of other institutional and ambulatory delivery settings.
> Congress should:
>
> > Designate the NFHQMR (now the NQF) as the entity responsible for promulgating and maintaining a core set of reporting standards to be used by states,
> > Require all health care organizations to report standardized information on a defined list of adverse events.

In addition, recommendation 5.1 stated that Congress should fund this reporting system and create a Center of Patient Safety that would share information and expertise to improve patient safety and reduce adverse events.[4]

"Consumer Reports" for Health Care

Because progress on reducing adverse events is moving slowly and error analysis is poorly shared across hospitals, the health care community, in partnership with safety organizations (such as those discussed previously) and consumer patient safety groups should consider the creation of a "consumer reports" type of publication to evaluate hospitals.

Researchers at the University of Missouri Health Care found that one of the key barriers to improving patient safety is "the silo approach to data collection, reporting and resolution of adverse events. For example, the events reported by patients concerning quality of care or patient safety could not be linked to an incident report filed by a nurse or to a review carried out by clinical departments [physician peer review] . . . therefore, multiple areas were addressing the same incident without coordination of efforts. The disparate nature of these paper-based systems and their inability to be linked ensured that few systematic prevention activities were undertaken."[5]

Scales of Improvement on Hospital Error Reductions

Creating a hospital consumer reports type of publication requires the consideration of a number of key steps. First, the consumer reports should consist of two key scales: a hospital's rating for the prevention of serious injuries and deaths compared to "like hospitals," and a scale that measures a hospital's progress toward improving patient safety. These adverse events would need precise definitions and begin with a small number, first focusing data analysis on the highest-risk errors known to hospitals, such as restraint deaths, wrong-site surgeries, and potassium overdoses. Specific patient case information would not be released.

Second, as discussed previously, there is a need for a centralized, standardized, and mandatory data depository for reporting hospital medical errors. In conjunction with current organizations like the NQF, analysis and data reports could be created at state levels.

Immunity from Punishment for Reporting Errors

Hospitals that participate in any federal or state data depository must receive immunity from fines, punishment, regulatory agency inspections, and surveys. This immunity would come with set principles for reporting, for example, the hospital must complete a medical error report and root cause analysis and submit it to the data depository within 30 days of the adverse event. If the submission occurs within the specified time frame, then punitive immunity should be granted to the hospital—with no exceptions.

Think about the ramifications had such a data depository been present after the first 12 deaths from injections of concentrated potassium. Since the early root cause analyses on mistaken injections showed that potassium errors occurred because vials were freely available on patient care units and that the highly concentrated solutions were easily being given to patients because they looked like other drugs (particularly Lasix), sharing these root causes early might have saved lives. What if, in 1996, these common causes had been mandated to be shared among hospital leaders? Would baby Gianni be alive today?

Granted, the alerts about lethal overdoses of potassium were shared because of the efforts of valuable organizations like the Institute for Safe Medication Practices, and many hospitals responded to the dangers; nevertheless, there were no mandates to remove the concentrated solutions until January 1, 2003. It should never have taken seven years to mandate this safety practice throughout all U.S. hospitals. Even though many hospitals had the data, there was no centralized database or mandate to share preventive root cause analysis strategies.

Next, new legislation or an amendment to the Health Care Quality Improvement Act should be considered to protect individual patient-specific information. Even with patient-specific error protection, the public would see error rates and would be able to track those hospitals that are making progress toward reducing preventable adverse events. The Institute of Medicine supports this and made a recommendation about extending peer review protection to patient-specific medical error data. Freely opening up disclosure on individual cases poses great liability issues for hospitals; however, trends on safety improvements can help drive consumers and insurance companies to select safer hospitals. This creates competition among hospitals, which also drives improvements in safety.

Last, scales of measurement and definitions must be precise, easy to interpret, and consumer friendly. The definitions should consider ease of data collection and there should be considerations for hospitals with limited resources, including those with few human resources and antiquated data-collection systems. Private and government subsidies should be considered to assist hospitals in reporting and analyzing data.

Table 12.2
Sample Report for Consumers

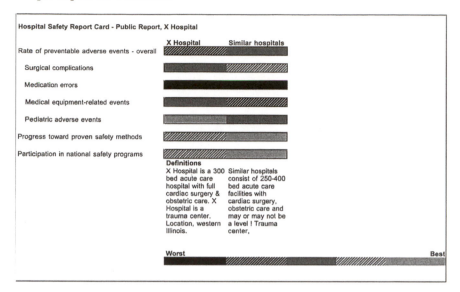

A consumer reports–type publication for U.S. hospitals could be published at least annually and perhaps as often as biannually or quarterly.

Consumer Reports magazine (Yonkers, New York) uses a graduated scale to measure consumer products including automobiles (inclusive of safety), electronics, computers, and other consumer items. Medical Artificial Intelligence (MEDai, Orlando, Florida), a company that provides quality data for hospitals, uses a "stoplight" approach for measuring outcomes on hospitals and physicians. A combination of these methodologies and other scientific measures could be created for the public so that people can reasonably know a hospital's performance on patient safety. The hospital-evaluation data published for consumers need to be just as clear and precise as the data that are available on purchasing automobiles and other consumer products.

Error Reduction Is Moving Too Slowly

The consumer reports–type model is simplistic, and more work would need to be done to develop meaningful information for consumers. However, currently little data are available to the public on medical errors or reduction efforts. Since the release of the IOM report, there has been scant evidence to show that hospitals have made progress in reducing preventable adverse events. Often a news-worthy event such as a child's untimely injury or death from a med-ical mistake will briefly stir up the media and the public. But once the flurry dies down, attention is diverted away from concern about med-ical errors. Yet, many health care consumers can relate stories of errors or inefficiencies that they have experienced.

An important objective of a consumer publication is to bring health care consumers into the process of a patient safety culture change through the monitoring of hospital trends. This will allow them to seek care at safer facilities, and it may also help them demand improvements as partners and gain knowledge, all while moving toward error reduction.

Change must be driven by a wider cross-section of the public than just those patients and families who have been forced to become hos-tile and angry because the system failed them. Those individuals will certainly help the cause, but changing health care should not be their sole responsibility. The knowledge that the data will provide will most likely guide the public to make safer choices and demand culture changes in health care.

Tips

Ask your hospital administration office if it posts quality or medical error data outcomes such as heart attack, stroke, surgery treatments, complications, and death rates on the hospital's Web site. If not, why not?

If you need surgery, ask your hospital how many cases of your type of surgery it performs each year. Ask for an outcome rate on complica-tions and death with this procedure.

When considering surgery, ask your surgeon how many of the same type of surgeries he or she has performed. Ask what your surgeon's complication rates are.

When considering surgery, ask the hospital what its surgical site infection rate is for your type of surgery.

When considering surgery, ask your surgeon what his or her surgical site infection rate is for your type of surgery.

To find out about the complication and death rates for surgery, call your hospital administration office or the quality department. The general staff will not know.

To find out about surgical site infections, call your hospital adminis-tration office or the infection control program. The general staff will not know.

A Little Assistance

In the 2003 federal budget, President Bush devoted attention to the dilemma of medical errors and patient safety. He proposed $10 million in new federal funding for programs that focus on reducing medical errors. Of the $10 million, $5 million was targeted for the Agency for Healthcare Research and Quality (AHRQ), which already has a $60 million budget to improve health care. The other $5 million was slated for the Federal Drug Administration to focus on error reports of injuries and deaths that occur during the use of FDA-approved medical equipment and drugs. The additional money will be used for training experts who can guide the implementation of proven but underused technologies that focus on patient safety. Much more needs to be done to address the urgent problem of medical harm. In the United States, given that more people die from adverse events in hospitals than die from automobile accidents, significant discussion needs to take place among legislative leaders on dollars for redesigning safer, "crash-worthy" hospital systems.

Someone Spoke Up

A pharmaceutical representative spotted stark similarities between two different drugs. The packaging and labels were the same color, with similar printing and type size, yet the medications themselves were very dissimilar. A mix-up could easily result in a patient's death.

One medication was a paralyzing agent that would instantly stop a patient's breathing. The other was to control high blood pressure. Should a patient with high blood pressure be given the paralyzing drug by mistake, the chance of death was likely. The pharmaceutical representative saw this danger and reported it to the company. The manufacturer changed the labeling. The representative should receive a reward or incentive for this important finding.

Like this pharmaceutical representative, consumers or any patient can report the same types of dangers.

Incentives and Monetary Awards

Awards—perhaps given by government and private foundations—should be considered for consumers and health care personnel who display leadership in identifying health care dangers and are role models for patient safety improvements. Scholarships for these individuals or their families are a possibility. Hospitals that lead the industry in patient safety should also be eligible for grants, such as private or public funds for technology upgrades and proven patient safety enhancements.

Several such awards and grants are currently available, but the competition for them is very tough. Recently, one hospital patient safety award had over 80 applicants the day it was announced. Grants should include dollars for creating community and patient partnership groups focused on patient safety. Simple, non-labor-intensive criteria for receiving grants and awards need to be in place. Many health care grants require time-consuming documentation of criteria.

Were the Patients Asked?

BETTY

In a Florida outpatient surgery suite in May 2001, Betty Weier, age 69, underwent surgery to repair her left Achilles tendon. To be certain that the correct leg was operated on, the word "no" was marked on her right foot. The surgeon came in to look at the foot. Betty was lying faceup and had just received her sedation from the anesthesiologist. The surgeon commented, "This is a good way to identify the leg."

The surgeon left the room to scrub for the surgery. He returned and began the procedure. After making the incision into the ankle, he saw the tendon and said, "This tendon looks fine." He asked the nurse to check the films. To the horror of both the surgeon and nurse, the doctor was operating on the wrong leg. Betty had been flipped over onto her stomach when the surgeon left the room to scrub.

Betty's good leg was stitched up, and the surgeon proceeded to operate on the correct leg. The surgeon apologized to Betty and her husband; however, she had two wounds to recover from. She later brought legal action against the surgeon.[6]

Marking Surgical Sites

Before January 2003, only 60 percent of orthopedic surgeons routinely marked surgical sites before an operation. However, in 1997 the American Academy of Orthopedic Surgeons started a program called "Sign Your Site." The intent of the program was to ensure that the correct surgery was done at the correct site and on the correct side. Since January 1, 2003, surgical sides and sites are required to be marked in accredited hospitals as the result of a mandate from JCAHO.

Surprisingly, almost all of the new processes related to the practice of marking surgical sites were put into place without input from former surgical patients. Physicians, nurses, quality leaders, and other clinicians all planned the new mandatory marking, discussing the best type of markers, when to mark, what to mark, and how to mark, and the new policies were put into place.

Perhaps asking former patients for their suggestions will assist in preventing some errors that have not yet been uncovered with the new mandates and practices. Hospital professionals will not know the benefits, or risks, of patient affiliations for safety until those partnerships are in place.

Mandate Human Factors Engineering

Human factors engineering (HFE) as discussed earlier should be mandated proactively into new hospital system design and redesign, much as the FDA is doing with medical devices. More research is necessary because little use of HFE practice currently exists.

Utilize More Disclosure

A study in the *Journal of the American Medical Association* on February 26, 2003 reviewed the work of researchers at Washington University School of Medicine who consulted focus groups with patients and professionals to get input on disclosure. Patients clearly expressed that they wanted to know if a mistake happened and how it could have been prevented. The patients also wanted an apology.[7] Increased disclosure by both hospitals and physicians is needed. As with any service, when errors occur, consumers want acknowledgment of the incident, not concealment of the facts. The practice of disclosure is simply ethical and decent. In addition, early studies in humanistic risk management have shown that disclosure to patients is beneficial. A transition from traditional risk management to a more compassionate model needs further consideration and research.

Patient Error-Prevention Surveys

Hospitals frequently carry out patient satisfaction surveys assessing patients' experiences in the hospital or receiving outpatient services. The results of the surveys are analyzed and reported to the board, executives, and clinicians. Action plans based on the survey results are formulated and executed within the hospital units. In these surveys, there are occasionally a few limited questions about safety, none of which are extensive. Generally, hospital marketing departments steer away from strongly worded questions regarding potential medical errors. They are concerned that patients will be scared off by direct questions about medical errors.

An appropriately written error-assessment survey could be used to evaluate compliance with the JCAHO safety standards, gleaning valuable data from the patients' perspective. Some useful questions might be, "Did your nurse always check two forms of identification before giving you medicine?" or "Was the site of your surgery marked prior to surgery?" or "Were you informed about the reason for marking your surgical site?"

If hospitals asked questions like this and trended the results for each hospital unit, then safety improvements could be implemented as guided by the results. The implementation of a new JCAHO mandate does not guarantee that the practice is consistently being carried out. Additionally, other problem areas could be identified through the survey and the necessary corrective actions taken. By not collecting this type of survey information, hospitals are missing out on valuable patient views. The creation of such a survey would also allow multiple hospitals to compare common safety concerns with each other and work collectively toward solutions.

Incident Alerts for Patients during Hospitalization

Hospitals should consider implementing a different type of incident report, one that does not have such strong affiliation with traditional incident reports. The purpose of this report would be for patients to alert the hospital to potential risks that are not actually adverse events. Patients who see potential risks or near misses could report them on an alert form. In addition, these trends could also continue to be handled through hospital management and patient-relations departments, as they are currently.

Consumer Input to Sentinel Event Reviews

Hospitals might consider the use of consumers' participation in sentinel event reviews. This process would involve selecting a group of articulate, well-versed former patients to sit in with sentinel event review teams. The former patients would not be patients affected by that particular error, but they would be previous patients who have a unique perspective on hospital care—perhaps patients involved in former errors.

These chosen individuals would have to enter into a strict confidentiality agreement that was stringently enforced. If additional protection were afforded to the error data as proposed, then the consumer members would have to uphold the same protections as doctors and professionals. The programs could be voluntary, or perhaps small monetary compensation would be provided. JCAHO might consider this as a pilot program.

Still Writing after All These Years

A 70-year-old woman who was hospitalized required a narcotic called Dilaudid for pain. She had a pump that would gradually and consistently infuse her pain medication for consistent relief. A physician wrote an order for a solution of the Dilaudid. As he wrote the order, he mistakenly entered the infusion rate on the wrong line of the order sheet. He recognized his error and crossed out the line where the concentration had been placed. The doctor then initialed and circled his change so that it would be authenticated. He then wrote the dose for "Dilaudid 2 mg in 250 ml of normal saline."

The pharmacist received the order and interpreted the doctor's circled initials as a zero. He mixed 20 milligrams of the Dilaudid in 250 milliliters of normal saline. The solution was administered to the patient.

Later that evening another nurse discovered the error when she compared the bag to the original order. The medication was immediately discontinued. Fortunately for the patient, she suffered no harm; however, this amount of Dilaudid could have led to respiratory arrest.[8]

Immediate Elimination of Handwritten Orders

There is no reason for the practice of handwriting orders to continue until full computerization is implemented. Consumers must immediately start rejecting any prescription that they cannot read.

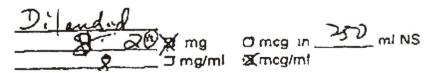

Two or twenty? Look closely at the zero. Institute for Safe Medication Practices.

Message

Can you read this? Institute for Safe Medication Practices.

The consumer has the right to ask the physician to legibly print another prescription. If even 20 percent of patients started to demand this practice tomorrow, it would change most likely the practice of illegible handwriting. Physicians would not want to be constantly rewriting prescriptions.

People can sometimes feel intimidated when doctors hand them a prescription. This is the very moment that the patient needs to speak up and reject the prescription, no matter how the doctor reacts. It is the patient's medicine, and it is the patient who will be the recipient of an error caused by bad handwriting.

Hospital medical executive committees should implement immediate revocation of handwritten and illegible physician orders. There is no reason—none whatsoever—that one more patient should be harmed because of this practice.

Recently, a registered nurse wrote to a state nursing publication with his comments about the 2003 JCAHO mandatory patient safety practices, which did not address handwritten orders:

> When I read, "Safety First, JCAHO introduces New Patient Safety Goals," my blood began to boil. As a nurse on a hospital medical floor, there is no doubt in my mind that the greatest potential threat to our patients' safety is physicians' poor handwriting.
>
> Three or four times each shift, physicians leave behind orders in utterly indecipherable scrawl. Nurses and pharmacists are left squinting at this gibberish and conferring among themselves to guess words, to figure out whether we have a 3 or 5 here or to divine the physician's reasonable intent since his penmanship is illegible.
>
> Besides the obvious danger of miscommunication about treatment and medications, vital patient care is delayed as we struggle to interpret the scribbling or wait for a physician to return the telephone page to clarify a stat scratched order.[9]

	or if temperature is ³ 101°F.		
	18. Blood culture x 2 for temperature > 101°F.		250 U/hep 8U pe hom
	19. Do limb circumferences Q_____hours		NO both
	20. Comments:		hold hepa for now
	hold Ohmoden		cancel haldol pt allepe

		NURSE'S SIGNATURE		PHYSIC~~_____~~
PHAR	NOTICO	X	Date / Time	

This order resulted in confusion between a "u" symbol and a zero. The order was for 250 units of heparin but was misread as 2500 units of heparin. Karin Berntsen.

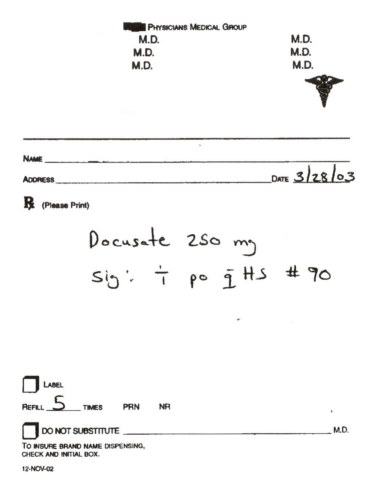

███ PHYSICIANS MEDICAL GROUP

M.D.   M.D.
M.D.   M.D.
M.D.   M.D.

NAME _____

ADDRESS _____ DATE **3/28/03**

℞ (Please Print)

Docusate 250 mg

Sig: ī po q̄ HS # 90

☐ LABEL

REFILL __5__ TIMES   PRN   NR

☐ DO NOT SUBSTITUTE _____ M.D.

TO INSURE BRAND NAME DISPENSING,
CHECK AND INITIAL BOX.

12-NOV-02

All of this physician's orders are printed legibly. Karin Berntsen.

Physicians are capable of writing prescriptions neatly, as displayed by the prescription of an actual doctor's order shown here. All of the prescriptions written by this doctor are legible.

Tips

When your doctor hands you a prescription, stop and read it. If you cannot read the writing, kindly ask the physician to reprint a neat prescription.

When your doctor hands you a prescription, carefully listen to the name of the medication and the instructions for taking it. If the information seems unclear to you, ask the doctor to repeat the name of the drug and the instructions until you fully understand them.

Simple Resources Provided to Patients

Few resources are available to guide patients through the complex health care system. Patients need direct and precise guides to help them with most health care services because each type of service is unique and poses some risks. Practical words of advice can help people be alert to and possibly decrease the chance of errors. Patient-focused resources should be available at all reading levels, along with audiovisual tools, and these materials should be available in multiple languages. Some resources are listed in appendix 2 of this book.

Tip

While in the hospital, if you do not understand a treatment, speak with your physician, your nurse, or both. If it is still not clear to you, or if you have other concerns, ask to speak with a nurse educator or case manager who may be able to give you additional information or perhaps a brochure on the treatment.

An Immediate Need

LITTLE TAYLOR

Shortly after midnight, Taylor McCormack, 14 months old, was rushed to the emergency department of a children's hospital. Her parents knew something was very wrong. When Taylor was born, she had needed a shunt to drain fluid from her brain.

Now the shunt had clotted off and Taylor needed urgent surgery to release the pressure from the fluid on her brain.

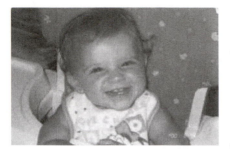

"I lived every parent's nightmare of losing a child and this is especially difficult because our child should be alive today, but because of medical errors, she is not." John J. McCormack.

The resident neurosurgeon ran critical blood tests as he tried desperately to tap the baby's shunt. Taylor's blood work was extremely abnormal—she had a high level of carbon dioxide, showing she was not getting enough oxygen to her brain. The attempts to drain the fluid were unsuccessful, and Taylor's condition deteriorated. The resident and staff desperately tried to page the on-call neurosurgeon, but they could not reach him. At 6:20 in the morning, little Taylor went into respiratory arrest and died. The neurosurgeon had placed his pager on vibrate and had fallen asleep.[10]

Hospitalized Children Often Experience Medical Injuries

In June 2004 the Agency for Healthcare Research and Quality released the largest study to date on the impact of injuries and errors on hospitalized children. The study examined 5.7 million patient medical records from 27 states. Children under the age of 19 were reviewed. The study identified 51,615 patient safety events involving children in hospitals in 2000. Children under 1 year old were at the highest risk for an adverse event. Medical injuries in children increased their length of stay, death rate, and hospital charges. On average, infections increased a child's length of stay in the hospital by 30 days and increased hospital charges by $121,000. The researchers also estimated the overall cost for these injuries at $1 billion. Based on these and other findings, there is clearly an urgent need to develop solutions to the problem of medical harm in children.[11]

The results of a study performed by the Center for Health Services and Clinical Research, Children's Research Institute, and the Children's National Medical Center found that hospital-related medical errors among hospitalized children ranged between 1.8 and 3 percent. Error rates were lower in 1988 than they were during each of the years 1991, 1994, and 1997, showing an increasing prevalence of medical errors. The study also found that special-needs children were at a higher risk for errors; however, it was clear that errors in children are underreported and that more research is urgently needed in this area.[12]

Children's Medical Error Prevention Foundation

A subsidiary foundation needs to be created with the sole intent of focusing immediate efforts on medical error prevention in children. A children's foundation, for example, could be established under the charter of one of the currently existing patient safety organizations or foundations.

The express mission of such a children's organization would be to implement an urgent program that would focus on immediately stopping medical errors in children. Critical areas such as medication administration, equipment failures, anesthesia, and surgical problems in pediatric and newborn populations would first be addressed. Children and infants are too young and too susceptible to medical errors to wait for the overall culture of patient safety to be reestablished. Just within the contents of this book, more than 15 children were harmed or killed by medical errors. This does not take into consideration the dozens of children's cases that were researched but excluded from the text.

Attention on children alone is enough to mandate swift improvements in patient safety. Although every life is critical, children's lives are certainly the most momentous. Government funding should be directed at the creation of a children's foundation for hospital error prevention in the next federal budget. Private funding can start immediately.

In 2001, the American Academy of Pediatrics took a clear stand on supporting the IOM and setting in place principles to promote patient safety in children. The academy and its members are committed to improving the health care system to provide the best and safest health care for infants, children, adolescents, and young adults. A set of principles was established to guide the profession in designing a health care system that maximizes quality of care and minimizes medical errors through identification and resolution. This set of principles provides direction on setting up processes to identify and learn from errors, developing performance standards and expectations for safety, and promoting leadership and knowledge.[13]

Taylor's Law

The physicians involved in Taylor's case were brought before the Massachusetts Board of Registration in Medicine for disciplinary actions; however, Taylor's parents, John and Catherine McCormack, were denied access to the proceedings. In May 2004 a new law was enacted in Massachusetts that allows patients and families access to disciplinary hearings against physicians. John McCormack, a police officer, fought hard for this legislation. The bill, brought forward by state Senator Therese Murray, allows families and patients to make victim impact statements at the disciplinary hearing. It also allows for letters of reprimand against physicians to be posted on the state board's Web site. Massachusetts is the first state to provide specific profiles on its Web site with the intention of helping patients make informed health care decisions.[14]

Tips

To see profiles of Massachusetts physicians, log on to http://profiles. massmedboard.org/Profiles/MA-Physician-Profile-Find-Doctor.asp.

You are your child's best advocate for safety. Ask questions, speak up, and get all the facts before you authorize treatment for your child.

If you are uncertain about a recommended treatment, seek a second opinion.

Use available resources for gaining knowledge, including the American Academy of Pediatrics Web site, "You and Your Family." Log on to http://www.aap.org/family/.

Contact your local children's hospital to obtain more information regarding care for your child.

Recommendations on Safety

The IOM has clearly set the stage for patient safety as a top priority in health care. The IOM's recommendation 7.2 states, "Performance standards and expectations for health care professionals should focus greater attention on patient safety." The IOM report further recommended:

Professional societies should make a visible commitment to patient safety by establishing a permanent committee dedicated to safety improvements with the following intents: 1) develop a curriculum on patient safety..., 2) disseminate information on patient safety..., 3) recognize the importance of patient safety in practice guidelines. . . , 4) develop community based initiatives for reporting and analyzing errors. . . , and 5) collaborate with professional societies and disciplines on the professional's role in patient safety.[15]

The American Medical Association (AMA) took a supportive stand in conjunction with the IOM report and created additional recommendations on patient safety. The IOM and the American Medical Association both support the concept of collecting more data on standardized medical errors.

Additionally, Dr. Kenneth Kizer testified before Congress in support of collecting and sharing further data on medical errors:

At present, medical errors are grossly under-reported, and there is extremely limited data about their occurrence. Creating an error data collection system is essential to the success of efforts to reduce their occurrence. Likewise, sharing information about errors with frontline clinicians is needed to further their understanding of the issues, as well as to promote collaboration and a sense of shared mission.

The AMA strongly supports the need for increased research on medical errors. Their recommendation states:

Conduct research that spans the entire scope of health service delivery, including hospital and ambulatory care and surgical procedures that are moving from medical centers to freestanding outpatient surgery clinics and doctors' offices, and reach from individual doctors and other providers to top management and governing bodies of health care institutions.[16]

The American Medical Association made these additional recommendations at its summit on patient safety:

Examine safety-engineering systems at the National Aeronautics and Space Administration and the airline industry.

Identify new legislation to extend confidentiality protections to institutions that sponsor and conduct research promoting learning from adverse events and errors.

Examine human factors, cultures and working environments within the nation's health care system.

Examine technology in health care, both as a tool for improving patient safety and as a factor in causing medical errors.

Evaluate market-based disincentives, including the increasing cost pressures and administrative burdens on hospitals and physicians.

Find the most effective communication tools for installing "best prac-tices" and increasing the knowledge bases of consumers and providers.

Identify the most effective continuing education alternatives for physi-cians and nurses to keep current on advances in their professions.[17]

AMA chair-elect Timothy T. Flaherty testified at the National Summit on Medical Errors and Patient Safety Research: "Patients have the right to expect their care will be provided in a culture of patient safety. Valid research is critical. Interventions must be non-punitive in nature and oriented to learning. We can change physician behavior through incident reporting. Near misses can be more impor-tant than adverse incidents. Voluntary and non-punitive reporting and analyses of 'near-misses' can lead to prevention of adverse inci-dents that must be reported."[18]

Michael R. Cohen, president of the Institute for Safe Medication Practices, agreed that research was critical; however, the research should not delay the implementation of evidence-based interventions for medical error reduction. He said, "Every day, there is clear evi-dence that another tragic medication error could have been prevented if knowledge had been transformed into action."[19]

Lastly, Dr. Kizer addressed Congress on the need for a culture of patient safety:

A number of characteristics define a healthcare culture of safety. For example, in a culture of safety there is open acknowledgment that mod-ern healthcare is a high-risk activity and that everyone in healthcare has a responsibility for risk reduction and error prevention. Errors are recognized and valued as opportunities for improvement, and there is a non-punitive and safe environment in which errors can be learned from. There is honest and open communication about safety issues with well-known mechanisms for reporting and learning from errors, and confidentiality of information. Likewise, in a culture of safety there are mechanisms for restitution and compensation for injuries that result from errors, and clear organizational commitment, structure and accountability for safety improvement.[20]

Patient Safety and Public Health Legislation

Patient Safety and Quality Improvement Act—HR 663

This bill, passed in the House of Representatives (HR) by a vote of 418 to 6, authorizes the secretary to establish patient safety organi-zations (PSO) to voluntarily collect and analyze confidential information on medical mistakes by health care providers. The bill was sponsored by Florida Representative Michael Bilirakis.

Patient and Physician Safety and Protection Act of 2003— HR 1228

This bill, introduced in March 2003, relates to residents' work hours currently under consideration. The purpose of this bill is to amend the Social Security Act to reduce the work hours and increase the supervision of resident physicians to ensure the safety of patients and the resident physicians themselves. The bill would require federal regulators from the Department of Health Services to handle all complaints of violations that arise from residents who report that their programs are in violation of the requirements on working hours for certain members of the medical staff and postgraduate trainees. This bill has been referred to the subcommittee of health. Its sponsor is Michigan Representative John Conyers, Jr.

Patient Safety Act of 2001—HR 1804 / S 863

This bill, introduced in May 2001 and cosponsored in the House and Senate (S), requires Medicare providers to publicly disclose their staffing and performance to promote improved consumer information and choice. The sponsors are New York Representative Maurice Hinchey and Nevada Senator Harry Reid.

Patient Safety and Healthcare Whistleblower Protection Act of 2001—HR 2340

This bill, if passed into law, would prohibit discrimination or retaliation against health care workers who report unsafe conditions and practices that impact on patient care. It is sponsored by Florida Representative Mark Foley.

Nursing Home Quality Protection Act of 2001—HR 2677

This bill, introduced in July 2001, amends title XIX of the Social Security Act to improve the quality of care furnished in nursing homes by improving nurse staff ratios, disclosing performance on the Internet, and more stringent quality improvement monitoring. The sponsor is California Representative Henry A. Waxman.

Medication Errors Reduction Act of 2001—HR 3992

This bill establishes an informatics grant program for hospitals and skilled nursing facilities to encourage providers to make major information technology advances by using medical information technology. An advisory board will develop and disseminate standards for the electronic sharing of medical information. It is sponsored by New York Representative Amo Houghton.

Safe Nursing and Patient Care Act—HR 745 / S 373

This bill, introduced in February 2003, amends the Social Security Act to provide for patient protection by limiting the number of mandatory overtime hours a nurse may be required to work for providers of services to which payments are made under the Medicare program. The sponsors are Massachusetts Senator Edward Kennedy and California Representative Fortney Stark.[21]

Tips

To learn more about patient safety legislation, contact the Centers for Disease Control at (202) 690-8598.

Patient safety legislative efforts have started over the last three years. It is important to contact your state representatives in support of these and other legislative proposals.

Changing a Culture

All the leading professional organizations and health care leaders have stood firm on the principle of creating an entirely new culture of patient safety. The dilemma of medical errors is not a temporary fad for health care. Change requires a fundamental shift in the direction and customs of the health care community and in the practice of medicine. This tremendous shift will not come without the partnership of an informed public that says, "Enough is enough; we must stop patient harm." Just as the airline industry has made marked improvements in safety, to the point where consumers feel more confident in the mechanics of airline safety, health care leaders, in partnership with consumers, must now create the same level of perceived safety in health care.

CHAPTER 13

HOSPITALS ON THE MEND

I solemnly pledge myself before God and the presence of this assembly to pass my life in purity and to practice my profession faithfully.

I will abstain from whatever is deleterious and mischievous and will not take or knowingly administer any harmful drug.

I will do all in my power to maintain and elevate the standard of my profession and will hold in confidence all personal matters committed to my keeping and all family affairs coming to my knowledge in the practice of my calling.

With loyalty I will aid the physician and devote myself to the welfare of those committed to my care.

—Pledge of Florence Nightingale

Hospital leaders took the Institute of Medicine's report "To Err Is Human" seriously. Many of them had witnessed, firsthand and for too long, patient harm. There was a strong sense of relief among these leaders that someone had finally substantiated the suspicions that the leaders previously recognized: that too many patients were being harmed. Yes, the leaders were aware that U.S. hospitals provide the best health care in the world, and they could tell countless positive stories about patients whose lives had been saved and vastly improved. Even so, beneath the surface was the fear of harming patients with misaligned systems and processes that were originally designed to help. Once the IOM research supported the error factor, hospitals were ready to begin safety improvements.

In addition to the hospitals' actions, the Healthcare Research and Quality Act was enacted in 1999. The purpose of this legislation was to establish the Agency for Healthcare Research and Quality (AHRQ), an agency of the Department of Health and Human Services. AHRQ is responsible for supporting research intended to improve health care quality, improve patient safety, decrease medical errors, reduce health care costs, and improve patient access to key medical services. The agency uses evidence-based research to assist health care decision makers and professionals to make more informed decisions about quality and safety.[1] AHRQ provides grants for various programs to enhance quality, safety, and education.

Hospital Changes

Hospitals began by formulating strategic plans for safety. Determining where to begin, however, was an overwhelming task. Generally, the planning was carried out by hospital executives, physicians, and the quality, risk, and environmental safety leaders who were already in place. Patient safety plans were written based on the recommendations from the IOM and other professional sources. Patient safety officers, some at the executive level, were assigned to head up the planning and implementation of safety.

Leaders' Patient Safety Education

The first objective was to bring the issues of medical errors to light among professionals and health care leaders. Publicity was going forward from the IOM report, but the facts surrounding medical and medication errors needed to reach every level of the organization. In truth, there was little shock over the magnitude of the problem, such as the fact that 44,000 to 98,000 patients died each year and many more patients were injured. A few studies tried to counter the volume of patients harmed, but these were not well received by the medical community.

Large national conferences began to take place, and hospitals committed resources to send leaders and employees to key educational sessions on safety. Internationally, summits were held. Medical errors are as extensive in western European hospitals, Australia, and New Zealand as they are in the United States. Leaders began to look for ways to share common ideas and strategies across hospitals and health care systems to improve patient safety. E-mail Listserves enabled professionals to share common concerns and safety practices.

Medication Safety for Patients

Improvements in medication safety were a launching point for scores of hospitals. Pharmacists and nurses knew for too long the dangers of medication errors. Collectively, pharmacists took a leadership role in initiating the culture change for patient safety. The work of the Institute for Safe Medication Practices was available to give the pharmaceutical industry valuable tools for preventing errors.

In 1999, the ISMP conducted an extensive professional survey to identify high-risk areas for medication errors. The survey results were shared across hospitals and on the ISMP Web site.[2]

Survey results showed some dangerous practices, such as use of nonstandard abbreviations, unsafe drug storage, and underuse of protocols for high-risk medications like chemotherapy administration. Improvements included better lighting in preparation areas, increased standardization, implementation of protocols, and education for pharmacy staff within hospitals. One practice that some hospitals have implemented is the use of a safe medication practice pharmacist, whose sole job is focused on medication error prevention.

Tips

Know your medications. Ask to see the medicines before you take them. Many medications come in individual packages known as unit doses. Before they are removed from their packaging, ask the nurse to bring your medicines in their original package so you can read the amount, drug, and dose. When you are in the hospital, be certain to learn about every medicine that you are given. What is it for, what is the dose, what is the administration route, and what are the side effects? They are your medicines, so be your own best advocate in understanding how they work.

Effective January 1, 2003, all JCAHO-accredited hospitals must have an approved list of acceptable abbreviations. Also included on this list are abbreviations not to use. Ask the health care professionals caring for you if they know about the abbreviation list.

A National Health Information System

In 2003 the IOM released a third report on the need for a national health information system that expands across hospitals, doctors' offices, and nursing homes. The report, *Patient Safety: Achieving a New Standard for Care* (National Academy Press), calls for the federal government to fund and develop national data standards. No doubt this comes as a result of the complex problem of medical errors and the lack of consistent data for creating feasible and standardized solutions that have been discussed throughout this text.

Members of the IOM Committee for Data Standards for Patient Safety outlined that Congress should authorize the Department of Health and Human Services to promote partnerships to develop standardized data. Hospitals working to solve the problem of medical errors will no doubt be affected if such authorization is granted.[3]

Physician Patient Safety Education

Physician education programs and national conferences shifted attention to the issues of patient safety. The American Academy of Family Physicians established the Center for Evaluation and Research in Patient Safety in Primary Care. The center's goal is to improve the safety and quality of medical care in family practice and primary care settings. The center was funded in part by a grant from the Agency for Healthcare Research and Quality. Research on medical errors is greatly needed in outpatient settings such as doctors' offices and clinics. Medical errors appear to be underreported in these settings.

Nurses' Commitment to Safety

No professional has taken the IOM report more seriously than nurses. Nurses have witnessed harm for too long, and often they are caught up in latent conditions that lead to medical errors. Nurses are responsible under their license to refuse any order that is dangerous for the patient. There are countless unreported incidents, where nurses have been the sole barrier in stopping patient harm. Professional nursing organizations have taken steps to enhance nursing education on error prevention, improve system designs, lead patient safety programs, and promote research in safety. However, much more needs to be done to address issues of nursing shortages and staffing ratios. Legislation efforts continue that enhance the nurse-to-patient ratio to improve safety.

Nurse-to-Patient Ratios

Nurse-to-patient ratio is defined as the number of nurses assigned to care for a particular number of patients in a unit of a hospital or skilled nursing facility. Generally, health care facility administrations set nurse-to-patient ratios based on the intensity of services provided to patients. For example, an intensive care unit may a set ratio of 1:2, 1 nurse for 2 patients; a medical unit may set a ratio of 1:6, 1 nurse for 6 patients; and a skilled nursing facility may set a ratio of 1:15, 1 nurse to 15 patients. A 2004 report from the Institute of Medicine, "Keeping Patients Safe, Transforming the Work Environment of Nurses,"[4] concluded that a consistent finding from recent studies done on nurse-to-patient ratios showed that worse staffing ratios (more patients per nurse) were associated with higher rates of non-fatal adverse events, including nosocomial infections, pressure ulcers, and cardiac and respiratory failures.

Over the last five years, there have been efforts by consumer groups, nursing organizations, and labor unions to initiate legislation to mandate improved nurse-to-patient ratios. California was the first state to propose such legislation, but to date this legislation has not been enacted. Because no study or group of studies can confirm the exact ratio that will improve patient safety and decrease adverse events, it is a challenge to set an exact ratio for hospitals and skilled nursing facilities by units. The experience and quality of nursing staffs can impact patient safety, in addition to the number of allied personnel, such as certified nurses' aides who provide the majority of care in nursing homes. Nurses who feel the pressure of busy hospital units, increasing intensity of care provided, and "sicker patients" feel that improved nurse-to-patient ratios will help dispel nurse burnout, attract more nurses to work within hospitals, and avoid medical errors. Mandating ratios will most likely increase the cost to health care organizations and may be difficult to comply with due to the nursing shortage. Yet, if improved nurse-to-patient ratios enhances safety, clearly there may be a significant cost savings over time. Much more research needs to continue in this area.

Tip

To learn more about the proposed legislation from the California Department of Health Services on nurse-to-patient ratios, log on to http://www.applications.dhs.ca.gov/regulations/.

Centers for Patient Safety

A growing focus on community-based safety solutions is reflected in the creation of patient safety centers. In 1999, Pittsburgh was the first city to start such a coalition, engaging over 75 professional and community leaders. The coalition formed a charter to improve quality, reduce errors, and control health care costs. The collaborative set out to eliminate medication errors and hospital-acquired infections in southwest Pennsylvania hospitals.[5]

In San Diego, the San Diego Center for Patient Safety (SDCPS) is a collaborative effort between the Veterans Affairs (VA) San Diego Healthcare System and University of California at San Diego (UCSD) Health Sciences.[6] The center was started by Matthew Weingar, who has authored work on human factors engineering. The primary objectives of the SDCPS are the following:

To build and educate a multidisciplinary collaborative research team to study critical issues in patient safety in a variety of health care settings, from operating rooms to nursing homes.

To utilize the Standardized Encounter technique as a research tool to identify critical patient safety issues, develop safety improvements to prevent errors.

To develop Patient Safety Laboratories for both real and simulated training and research in a range of clinical care environments. The team plans to create a Realistic Patient Simulation environment that recreates the complexity of the operating room, intensive care unit or emergency room, using a sophisticated computer-controlled mannequin that mimics patient responses to medical treatment, from blood pressure and heart rate to reaction to pain.

To develop a website, training programs, and patient safety course materials to assist clinicians and patients to learn about and implement new safety techniques.[7]

In addition, the center offers a Web link for patients. This link provides patient educational resources for the prevention of medical and medication errors.

Tip

To view the San Diego Center for Patient Safety Web site, log on to http://cybermed.ucsd.edu/SDCPS/images/Intro_to_SDCPS.pdf.

Consumer Health Care Literacy

Generally, the more informed people are about their injury, illness, disease, and course of treatment as well as the application of that knowledge, the better the chances for good outcomes. Health care literacy is a central issue in the United States. Although more knowledge is critical to every population, a fact sheet from the Center for Health Care Strategies (CHCS) states that, "the older people, non-whites, those of low income and immigrants are disproportionately more likely to have trouble reading and understanding health related information."

According to a survey conducted by the 1992 National Adult Literacy Survey, 75 percent of Americans who reported having a long-term illness (six months or longer) had limited literacy.[8] Literacy issues are an important factor in the design of health care education and safety information. Not only should patient-education material about health-related illnesses be available in a range of reading levels, so should information about medical error prevention. Even simple materials for children could be helpful. Young children with chronic illnesses learn and adapt to new information very quickly. Providing them with safety ideas as well as the simple tools that enable them to speak up should be considered in pediatrics circles.

Healthy People 2010

The organization Healthy People 2010, which operates under the auspices of the Department of Health and Human Services, has focused on community-based improvements in prevention, disease control, and patient access. The organization challenges consumers, communities, and professionals to take steps toward promoting good health and enhancing life expectancy.[9]

One aim of the program is to increase health care literacy among populations with low literacy. Safety education is an area that is important for every group of citizens, particularly those who may be at higher risk for error because of their inability to read and interpret complicated prescriptions and instructions.

Tip

For more information about Healthy People 2010, log on to its Web site at http://www.healthypeople.gov/default.htm.

Take Caution Even with New Tools

As health care slowly moves toward the implementation of new electronic systems and advanced technologies, health care workers must use caution when using those new tools. Although the technologies offer advanced safety features, there are still unseen dangers, as demonstrated in the following case study. The fundamental principles of sound patient care must always remain constant.

Advances in Health Care: The Domino Effect

MRS. K

Staying with the Basics: Listening to the Patient

In North Carolina, Mrs. K entered the hospital at 9:00 P.M. in early labor to deliver her third child. Her water had broken at home and her labor had begun that afternoon.

Her first child had been born by emergency C-section, and her second baby was delivered by a successful vaginal birth after cesarean (VBAC). An administration of pitocin was given, the labor progressed, and her cervix became fully dilated. The baby moved into a + 1 position, just below the mid-pelvis.

Mrs. K began to tell the nurses that her pain was unusual. The nurses checked the fetal monitor and repositioned Mrs. K. There was nothing abnormal on the monitor reading. Labor began to progress very slowly; the baby had not moved any farther down the birth canal.

Mrs. K started to become anxious. She told the nurses, "This pain is definitely different from my other labor." Again, the nurses evaluated the monitor and found nothing abnormal. They figured that the position of the baby was probably causing this "different" type of pain.

The hospital had implemented a network of direct-connect cell phones for the physicians. The nurses were confident that with this new phone technology they could reach the doctor quickly. The nurse taking care of Mrs. K connected directly with the obstetrician and updated him on the patient's progress. He asked about the monitor. The nurse said it was normal, but that Mrs. K was complaining of odd pain, even though the monitor and vital sign readings were fine. The nurse faxed copies of the monitor readings directly to the doctor.

It was 2:15 A.M. and it had been over three hours since Mrs. K began this stage of labor. The baby was still at a + 1 position. Mrs. K was now in significant pain and her heart rate was elevated. She continued to say that the pain was "very different." The nurse connected with the physician and he headed toward the hospital.

Immediately after the call to the obstetrician, Mrs. K felt a ripping pain in her abdomen, and the baby's heart rate dropped dangerously low. The staff rushed Mrs. K into the operating room just as the physician was arriving. The doctor performed an emergency C-section and discovered that Mrs. K's uterus had ruptured.

Mrs. K was bleeding profusely and went into shock. The baby was lethargic and had to be resuscitated. Mrs. K had an emergency hysterectomy and received several blood transfusions. Both mother and baby survived.

A later investigation revealed that the staff had depended too heavily on the technology and not on basic assessment skills and listening to the patient.

In retrospect, early in the event, Mrs. K's heart rate and blood pressure were beginning to elevate, an early sign of a physiological change. The changes were very subtle, and alone they did not seem significant. However, in light of the patient's anxiety and "unusual pain," the combination of elevated heart rate and blood pressure were a clue that something was wrong.

New safety technologies are advanced tools, but, as with any new field of study or state-of-the-art tools, there are still components that can lead to errors. The technology advances are excellent, but fundamental principles of caring for patients and hearing their needs must never be superseded by reliance on these technologies.

CHAPTER 14

WHAT YOU CAN DO TO PROTECT YOURSELF

Gain Knowledge Before You Need It

The importance of gaining knowledge about the risks of potential medical errors and system flaws has been thoroughly discussed throughout this text. However, it is beneficial, if possible, to gain this knowledge before health services are needed or before a sudden injury or illness occurs.

Selecting a Doctor

Selecting a doctor is one of the most important things a person can do to assure reliable care. Building a trust relationship with a competent physician can be the backbone of receiving good care. The old "sense of community" should again be established. When a bond can be formed between physician and patient and the doctor gets to know the patient—not unlike the traditional days of Marcus Welby or, for the younger crowd, Dr. Brown, the "Everwood physician," this doctor can be an excellent patient advocate.

No one factor can lead to an appropriate decision regarding the selection of a doctor. Multiple factors should be considered and balanced together for a final selection. Health plans provide a preselected list of physicians, but the choices can be overwhelming. One of the first areas to consider is a physician's reputation among his or her physician colleagues and other hospital professionals. Hospital staff members work regularly with doctors and are usually aware of a physician's clinical and interpersonal skills. Asking a trustworthy health care professional can be helpful as you gather other facts.

Physician referral centers, run by hospitals, can be a useful source of information. The center's information on doctors is based on contractual issues, although health plans do have access to some of the physicians' outcome data. Health plans use these data for contracting acceptable practitioners who are then listed in the referral center's data. Be aware that neither the general hospital staff nor the referral centers have access to peer review data or closed-case review outcomes.

Using board certification can be beneficial when it is factored in with other information. Be alert, however, that there are some excellent non–board certified doctors as well as board-certified physicians who are not competent practitioners.

Other factors to consider are the length of time a physician has been practicing and the number of procedures or treatments that he or she has performed in a specific area. Online data sources on physicians' ratings should be used in conjunction with other types of information. The online sources are helpful, but they do not have all the data and information on physicians, and they certainly do not have access to confidential information or the data that is in the National Practitioners Data Bank.

A friend's experience with a doctor is a subjective measure and should not be reason alone to select a doctor. Choosing a doctor should never be based on one piece of information such as a phone book or random selection of names.

If time allows, it can be beneficial to interview a physician. During the physician interview, ask questions about schooling, training, experience, board certification, and procedure and complications rates. A written list of questions is helpful and will keep the interview precise and to the point for both the doctor and the patient.

Referral to a Specialist

When you are referred to a specialist, use the same criteria as mentioned previously. The referral from the primary doctor does not have to be your only choice. Ask for several names and ask the doctor, "If you were needing this procedure or surgery, would you go to the physician you are referring me to?"

In selecting any physician, a patient's instinct and interaction when meeting the doctor is extremely important. If something seems out of place, listen to those feelings and continue to search out other options.

Selecting a Hospital

Depending on geographic location, a patient may face more limitations in the selection of a hospital than in the selection of a physician. In addition, where a patient's physician practices and health plan provider requirements may narrow the choice. If you can select among hospitals, it is essential to find out some key factors about each one. The closest hospital may not always be the best selection.

Pay attention if a hospital has a particularly poor reputation in the community. Struggling, low-quality hospitals often rapidly acquire such reputations. If you have friends, or friends of friends, who are reputable health care professionals, it is important to ask them for their opinions about the hospitals in your area. You can use the JCAHO Web site to evaluate JCAHO-accredited hospitals. This Web site allows users to review pertinent survey results. If a physician practices at more than one hospital, then seeking his or her opinion as to the better of the two is also helpful.

Tip

Check the JCAHO Web site to see your local hospital's accreditation score. Log on to http://www.jcaho.org/, then go to the section "General Public" and then click "Quality Check," "Consumers," and "Search by Organization." Here you can enter the name of your hospital.

Once Diagnosed

Once you have a diagnosis, you need to obtain professional health-related information. After giving you a diagnosis, a physician is obligated to provide information to help you understand your diagnosis, including a complete explanation regarding treatment options, diagnostic tests, and medications or procedures required to treat the condition. Aside from the physician's advice, you can seek counsel from specialized nurse educators or case managers. Many physicians and hospitals employ these specially trained nurses. Sometimes they are certified in a particular specialty, such as diabetes education, in addition to their nurses' training. These specialized nurses can provide a wealth of information, and for many diagnoses insurance will pay for your visits or classes.

Risk Factors

With a new diagnosis, a physician should explain the side effects and risks of any required treatments such as medications or surgery. The physician should take sufficient time to completely address the patient's concerns, particularly those related to new medication use. The American Medical Association provides recommendations for physicians on supplying medication advice to their patients: "The AMA encourages physicians to counsel their patients about their prescription medicines and, when appropriate, to supplement with written information; and supports the physician's role as the 'learned intermediary' about prescription drugs."[1]

If a person has a preexisting condition such as diabetes, asthma, or cardiac disease, physician and patient should thoroughly discuss the effects of the new diagnosis on the current illness. This discussion should include drug interactions between newly prescribed medicines and current medications.

Tip

Once you have been told you need surgery or specialized treatment, stop, listen, and clarify exactly what the doctor is telling you. Do not feel rushed or intimidated about the time this takes. This is your time to obtain all the details you need about surgery. *Never assume* any information; *stop and clarify the facts.*

Professional Organizations

Following a diagnosis, make no assumptions about any factor related to that diagnosis. If information is unclear, ask for clarification. Depending on the illness or injury, resources from professional organizations, such as the American Heart Association or the American Academy of Orthopedic Surgeons, are beneficial. Professional organizations, often through their Web sites, provide reliable information for the public, especially for common illnesses and injuries. Some of the Web sites explain universal risks and side effects associated with various treatments. These sources can be very helpful for patients trying to make informed decisions about a course of treatment.

WebMD

WebMD Health is an online organization whose purpose is to "blend award-winning expertise in medicine, journalism, health communication, and content creation to bring the best health information possible."[2] The combined resources, covering most areas of health care, represent the largest medical information service currently provided. In 2003 an average of 20 million users visited the WebMD Web site per month.[3]

Take Time

During nonemergency cases, never feel rushed into surgery or treatment options before you have obtained full information. After a diagnosis, your physician should explain who will be performing the treatments or surgery. It is also essential for patients to know what to expect if they select not to undertake the recommended course of action.

ROSA

Rosa, age 44, loved to work in her yard. She had raised her son and now had more time to grow special roses and plant vegetables in her garden. In recent years, Rosa's hands had become painful and were beginning to lock up at the joints. Rosa also felt extreme stiffness in her hands in the morning, after she had worked a long time in her garden the day before.

Rosa had a friend who had undergone wrist surgery for a fracture repair the previous year. Rosa decided to visit her friend's surgeon to see if he could help her with her hands. At the visit, the surgeon examined Rosa's hands and told her that she had Dupuytren's contracture, a condition in which the tendons in the hands begin to thicken and the hands contract. The surgeon said that he could surgically repair her hands. That day at the office, the doctor's staff scheduled surgery on her right hand for the following Monday. The staff said that six weeks later they would schedule surgery on the other hand. Rosa agreed, although she felt like everything was moving too quickly.

When Rosa went home she decided to read more about Dupuytren's contracture. She logged on to a professional orthopedic Web site. The more she read about her condition, the more uncomfortable she became with how fast the surgery had been scheduled. From what Rosa read, she was unsure about the diagnosis.

The disease was not common in Hispanic women, and it was found seven times more frequently in men. She also did not have any of the preexisting conditions that were common in people with Dupuytren's contracture, such as diabetes. Although Rosa's fingers were slightly curled and she had a great deal of pain, she did not feel as though her tendons were becoming thicker.

She decided she wanted to see another physician. Rosa's HMO allowed her to obtain a second opinion, and her health plan referred her to a local hospital's telephone referral center. She scheduled an appointment that week with one of the recommended doctors.

At her appointment, the doctor took a family history. Both Rosa's mother and grandmother had suffered from severe arthritis as they aged. The doctor ordered X-rays of both hands and reviewed the results while Rosa was there. He told her that she had progressing osteoarthritis and that he did not recommend surgery. He felt that surgery would not solve the problem, and in fact, the resulting scar tissue would make her hands worse. He wanted her to begin taking aspirin daily and to soak her hands in warm water twice a day. He also scheduled her to have hand splints made so she could wear them at night to help prevent the fingers from curling.

All of the new treatments worked well for Rosa, and she was able to continue tending to her beautiful garden.

Be the Squeaky Wheel

According to Boston University School of Public Health's Patient Rights Program, "Every competent adult patient has the legal right to decide whether to accept or reject any medical care—even emergency or life-saving care."[4]

It can be easy to feel intimidated by the atmosphere of time pressure and uncertainty as you are shuffled through the rush and chaos of a health care facility, hospital, or doctor's office. It appears that the professionals always know best and that their recommendations should be followed. Certainly, in many cases professional advice is sound and reliable; nonetheless, stopping, taking time to learn, asking for clarification, and most of all speaking up if you have any concerns are essential. The patient should not fear stopping the health care professional and asking for more information to make a decision.

Often, when an unexpected injury or sudden illness occurs, patients sense a desire to relinquish control to "someone who seems to know best." Certainly, there are times when a patient's life is in jeopardy and immediate decisions need to be made. Even in such cases, it is critical to stop and focus carefully on the facts at hand. Get as much information as is available and carefully work with the physicians and professionals to make the best decisions based on all the facts. If a recommendation seems out of place or unusual, ask to speak to another physician or professional to clarify the facts.

Bring a Family Member or Friend

Select a close, trustworthy family member or friend to bring with you to the doctor's office or health care setting. This is especially important when you are being admitted to the hospital. A family member or friend may think of questions that you may not remember. He can also help to write down information and clarify your questions at a later time.

Other Advocates

If a friend or family member is not available, or if privacy is a concern, the hospital can provide a patient advocate. Some community programs also provide this service, such as the ombudsperson groups discussed in chapter 10. If you need such an advocate, speak to a hospital representative who can help you contact an appropriate advocate.

Follow Up on Test Results

It is a patient's right to have access to his or her own health care information. At the time your physician orders one or more test(s), ask the doctor to mail you a copy of all the test results. For an X-ray or laboratory test, a copy of the dictated results can be sent.

At times a patient will undergo tests such as blood work or imaging studies and will not hear back about the results. Patients often assume that the test results are normal and that nothing out of the ordinary exists, believing they would receive a call if a test was abnormal. Always call the physician within a few days of the diagnostic test(s) and ask for the specific results. This is a key area in which patients must be persistent until they have received their test results, whether positive or negative.

Tip

Ask to receive copies of all diagnostic tests that you have completed. Start a health care folder and keep the test results in it.

Be sure to complete all the tests that your doctor has ordered. The physician needs all the specific tests in order to make an accurate diagnosis.

FRANK

Another Close Call

Frank Barrera, age 48, was told he had prostate cancer and that he needed to undergo surgery to remove his prostate gland. Frank was prepared for surgery. The IV was started and the operating room was ready. Before the surgery started, the phone rang. It was the pathology department. There had been an error. The pathology department had read the wrong slide. Frank did not have cancer.

"You can imagine it was like waking up from a bad dream," Barrera said. The mistake was caught just in time.[5]

Misdiagnosis and Inappropriate Treatment

It is difficult to determine exact figures on the pervasiveness of misdiagnosis. There is a public perception that misdiagnosis occurs frequently. In 1997, the National Patient Safety Foundation (NPSF) conducted a telephone survey of people's perception of medical errors. Forty-two percent of the respondents reported a medical mistake, and of that group, 40 percent said the error was related to a misdiagnosis or treatment error. Eight percent stated that this misdiagnosis is what caused the medical mistake. Many of the medical studies performed on misdiagnosis are specific to specialized areas, such as the emergency department or a specific diagnosis such as appendicitis. There are limited studies on the overall prevalence of misdiagnosis; yet, a large number of people can discuss significant anecdotal cases surrounding misdiagnosis. More large-scale studies on this should be undertaken.[6]

In a study published in the *New England Journal of Medicine* (24 July 2003), 7,000 medical records from 12 cities were reviewed, and researchers found that patients with diabetes were not appropriately treated 75 percent of the time and patients with heart disease did not have proper treatment up to 40 percent of the time. Much of the blame for these troublesome factors in treatment was attributed to poor systems involving paper records, missing information, and the large numbers of patients that physicians have to see in a short time. Obtaining the appropriate history of a patient's illness was challenging due to these outdated systems.[7] Although this is a significant study that includes more than misdiagnosis, there are no widespread studies that can confirm or deny the exact prevalence of misdiagnosis. Nevertheless, misdiagnosis does occur, and as a patient you should take every opportunity to try to give your physicians accurate information about your history and presenting symptoms.

Error in Diagnosis

Diagnostic tests are subject to three types of error: testing errors, system flaws, and human mistakes. Testing errors can be test results known as false positives or false negatives. An example of a false negative would be an X-ray of a bone that has a small fracture. When the films are read, the doctor interpreting the film misreads the results and does not see the fracture, hence reading the results as negative. This would be a missed fracture, or false negative.

In a laboratory, a patient might have a test done to check the function of his or her liver. The result comes back as abnormal, but the patient has no symptoms of liver disease. The test is repeated twice, and the patient's liver tests are normal. The first test would be a false positive. Certain medications can cause laboratory false negatives or false positives, so it is important to tell the doctor about all substances you are taking, including medications, over-the-counter products, vitamins, minerals, herbs, and supplements.

All newly introduced laboratory tests are researched for the rate of false positives and false negatives, and quality-control measures are put in place to try to avoid this. Laboratories are strictly regulated for quality control in an attempt to avoid any type of laboratory or human error. Quality steps are taken to coordinate work flows, and training is continually reinforced for laboratory personnel. When an error occurs, even a minor one, steps are often taken to avert similar future errors.

Yet system flaws or human factors can occur, and people need to be alert to this. For any serious diagnosis or tests that result in a significant treatment or surgery, such as an organ removal for cancer,[8] potent drug administration, or other major surgery, a second opinion should be sought and second pathology test obtained. A person diagnosed with cancer has every right to have tests repeated, even by a different physician and a different laboratory. Occasionally, even a third opinion or test is warranted.

Second Opinions and Second Tests

The American Medical Association encourages the use of second opinions: "Physicians should recommend that a patient obtain a second opinion whenever they believe it would be helpful in the care of the patient. When recommending a second opinion, physicians should explain the reasons for the recommendation and inform their patients that patients are free to choose a second opinion physician on their own or with the assistance of the first physician. Patients are also free to obtain second opinions on their own initiative, with or without their physician's knowledge."[9] The short period you have to wait to repeat a diagnostic pathology report or to see another doctor in a nonemergency situation is reasonable.

The following are additional conditions under which a person should consider obtaining a second opinion:

- When the first physician is not an expert with a specific disease
- When a patient is interested in undergoing a medical alternative that his or her doctor is not familiar with
- When a patient is not comfortable about the advice that has been provided

If a doctor becomes angry or resistant to a patient's wish for a second opinion, this should be taken as a warning sign, and a second opinion should definitely be sought.

Online Second Opinions

A few large hospitals, such as the Cleveland Clinic in Ohio, now offer online second opinions. However, these practices are new, and it is too early to determine the reliability of this service.

Tips

When seeing a doctor for new symptoms of an illness, tell the doctor all of your symptoms, even if they seem unimportant or embarrassing. Every piece of information you give the doctor will help him or her make a better scientific diagnosis.

Seek another opinion if you are uncomfortable with the recommended course of treatment.

Seek a second opinion if you have been given more than one treatment option for a diagnosis.

Obtain a second opinion if you are having trouble obtaining a diagnosis.

Seek a second opinion if you have been diagnosed with a serious illness such as cancer or a rare disease.

In most cases, Medicare will provide you with the option to obtain a second opinion. Call your health plan representative for details.

Talk with your doctor about seeking a second opinion. The American Medical Association encourages physicians to be cooperative with a patient's request for a second opinion.

Most HMOs and health plans allow for second opinions. Contact your health plan for details.

If your health plan denies a second opinion, ask it to explain the reason and put it in writing.

If your first and second doctors have differing opinions, Medicare will often allow for a third opinion. In the event this happens, call your Medicare representative and explain the situation.

Bedside Manner

Many people have said, "I will go only to a doctor with a good bedside manner." A physician's bedside manner is important; everyone wants to be treated cordially and with respect. Conversely, a physician may have the best bedside manner in the world, but he or she may be an incompetent practitioner. It is clearly preferable to put up with a doctor who is seemingly cold and unfriendly but has the best skill possible.

A Word about Surgeons

Hospital workers often wonder why surgeons have a certain type of personality. They are often described as irritable, rude, or even mean. These traits sometimes seem to be stronger in highly specialized physicians and surgeons. Though I do not wish to exonerate the behavior, surgeons are often perfectionists who have an overpowering need to be in control. These are not bad traits for a surgeon to have when she is cutting around the heart or performing other critical, life-and-death procedures. Perfectionism, taking charge, and being in control are needed in almost any surgery or critical procedure.

Although hospital staff members complain about these types of behavior from physicians, those select physicians are often the surgeons of choice for staff members when they or their family members need surgery. This does not justify throwing scalpels across the operating room or engaging in screaming fits, but it is important to understand that bedside manner is not everything. Looking for skill and expertise is far more important than a great bedside manner. Of course, you have truly found a jewel if you discover a physician with a great bedside manner as well as superb technical skills. Such practitioners certainly do exist.

Tip

Closely follow your doctor's orders after any type of surgery. Generally, getting up after routine surgery with the assistance of a professional can diminish the chance for some complications such as skin breakdown, breathing problems, and blood clots. Be sure, however, to follow your doctor's orders after any procedure.

A Word about Children

As discussed previously, children represent one of the most vulnerable populations within hospitals. They are susceptible to high doses of medicine because they have neither the body weight nor the physiological development to handle abnormal medication amounts or volumes. They are also too young to note abnormalities. Parents are the best advocates for their children when it comes to receiving health care. Most health care services provided to children are excellent and are supplied in a competent and caring manner. It is important, nonetheless, to be alert and proactive when children are receiving health care services.

Tips

Do not share another adult's or child's prescription under any circumstances.

Do not use old prescription medications to treat a new illness.

Always thoroughly and completely read the instructions for taking prescription and over-the-counter medications.

When giving medicines by spoon, be certain that you are not confusing teaspoon and tablespoon. A tablespoon holds three times as much as a teaspoon. Carefully use the premarked cups that come with the medications, but be cautious, as the tsp and tbsp abbreviations look very similar. If you are uncertain, contact your pharmacist or physician.

Each time you administer medication to your child, check the bottle instructions for the right medicine, right dose, right route of administration, right time, and right child. It is easy to mix up your child's prescription medicines with yours or another child's. Bottles of prescriptions look the same and are easily confused with one another.

Never leave medicines within the reach of children, even if it is for just a few seconds or minutes. It takes only moments for a small child to ingest large volumes of medicines. Always secure medicines out of the reach of children.

If you are uncertain about any portion of the directions for administering a medication, contact your pharmacist or physician.

When filling new prescriptions for your child, always take part in the pharmacist consultation. Even if you have had the medicine in the past, the pharmacist can sometimes give you additional information that you did not know before. If your pharmacist does not offer you a session, ask for one.

Every time you pick up prescription refills, examine the medicine. If something looks different or if you have any questions or concerns, talk with the pharmacist. Make sure that you clearly understand what was said. If you are still uncertain when you get home, call your doctor.

When seeking treatment for a cold for you or your child, have a thorough discussion with your physician as to the true need for an antibiotic. Your child may truly need one; however, many colds are caused by viruses, and antibiotics are an ineffective treatment. Many physicians feel pressured by patients or parents to prescribe antibiotics. The overuse of antibiotics has contributed to the development of resistant organisms, such as MRSA. This is a growing and major problem and will become even more significant in the near future.

If you are given sample medicines in the doctor's office, check the dates to make sure the medicines have not expired. Read all the directions carefully. If you do not have directions, ask the doctor to write the directions down. If you do not understand the directions, confirm them with the doctor or nurse until everything is clear. You can also log on to the pharmaceutical manufacturer's Web site to obtain additional information on the medication.

Children in the Hospital

When a child is hospitalized, the experience is traumatic for both the child and the family. A temporary illness, an injury, or a chronic disease in a child poses many challenges for parents. The specially trained professionals in pediatric medicine are remarkable and attempt to make hospitalization go as smoothly as possible. Even so, it is critical that parents understand and participate in the entire course of treatment for any hospitalized child.

Tips

When your child is first admitted to the hospital, check all of the admitting papers very carefully to ensure they are accurate.

Make sure your child is weighed; do not use a previous weight or make a guess. Many medications are weight based, and it is critical to have an accurate weight.

For any procedure your child is undergoing, ask for the details of what will be done. Ask what medications and treatments will be used.

Read all consent forms in detail. Unless it is an emergency, never feel rushed when reading the paperwork. If you do not understand the information, ask for assistance.

For procedures or surgeries involving particular sides or sites of your child's body, confirm thoroughly the correct site and side with your physician and repeatedly with all members of the health care team. The JCAHO requires all accredited hospitals to mark surgery or procedure sites and sides. Carefully confirm the correct area with the physician and nurses performing the procedure or surgery.

A Word about Older Adults

As adults age, body functions begin to slow down. These changes can lead to diminished organ functions, memory loss, muscle weakness, immune system depression, and slower ability for the body to metabolize medications. Older adults should be constantly aware of the medications they are given, and they need to be cautious when started on new drugs. Work specifically with your doctors and nurses to review new and current medications. Any change in behavior or development of new symptoms should be reported immediately.

Medications are filtered and excreted by the body through either the kidneys or the liver, and if these organs have diminished function, then medications may not be cleared from the body correctly. Monitoring the effects of medications in older adults, people with liver or kidney disease, and people with preexisting conditions such as diabetes is extremely important. Also, being aware of interactions between medications is a particular concern in these populations.

Older people are susceptible to falls when they are hospitalized. Older adults may have a difficult time adjusting to hospital environments, and this becomes particularly worse at night, although problems can occur at any time. Older people are particularly prone to confusion when they awake during the night. They may not remember where they are. They should always be told, and the fact should be reinforced, not to get out of bed without help. Putting a large, bright sign in front of their bed may remind them that they are in the hospital and they need to call for help in getting out of bed. Repeatedly assure older patients that the call light stays near their reach. The call light has a tendency to be unintentionally moved by hospital workers. It needs to stay in close proximity to the patient.

Tips

After surgery, watch for early signs of confusion in your family member such as repeating questions, unaware of the surroundings or increasing agitation. These may be early signs of delirium. Report these changes to the nurse or physician immediately.

Do not use day-of-the-week travel pill containers. An older person who may have trouble discerning slight color variations can take the wrong pills.

Disabilities and Fall Risk

Hospital rooms are very small and very crowded. It is not uncommon for walkers, canes, and wheelchairs to get moved away from a patient's reach. It is particularly important that older adults, especially those who use walking aids, always ask for assistance when getting out of bed or moving about.

Tips

Clearly mark all of your walking aids with your name, your family's name, and your family's contact number.

When an older adult or any person is started on a new medication, *any* unusual side effects should be reported immediately.

For older persons as well as other patients, lost items such as eyeglasses and dentures is a common occurrence within hospitals. If you are admitted to the hospital or if you are having planned surgery, bring a small cosmetic or travel bag with you. Keep your valuable daily items such as eyeglasses and dentures in the bag. Clearly mark the bag with your name and phone number.

If you are admitted to the hospital and have high-value items with you such as credit cards, jewelry, or cash, ask your nurse to have these items checked into the hospital safe.

Other Special Patients

MR. HORDMEDKA

Bob Hordmedka entered a California hospital for an angiogram. Mr. Hordmedka had type 2 diabetes, and he had fasted the morning of the procedure as directed. Mr. Hordmedka suffered from sporadic episodes of low blood sugar. Sometimes when his blood sugar dropped too low, he would become combative due to the lack of glucose to his brain.

Mr. Hordmedka reminded the staff that he had diabetes and that he had not eaten that morning. He was given some sedation, and the hours began to tick by. His wife, Dawn, became concerned that too much time was passing. He continued to remind the staff about his diabetes and the fact that he had not eaten. They seemed to dismiss this.

Mr. Hordmedka was taken into the cath lab; it had now been 18 hours since he had eaten. Shortly after the procedure, he began to flail about convulsively. The staff called a restraint code on him, thinking the reaction was to the sedation, when in fact it was because of his low blood sugar. He was given glucose and revived.[10]

Diabetes

People with diabetes need to be especially diligent in monitoring their blood glucose and food intake during hospitalization. They should bring their own glucose meters and an ample supply of testing strips to the hospital.

A patient with diabetes who is admitted to the hospital should ask to speak with the diabetes nurse or a certified diabetes educator. This nurse can review with the patient his or her normal diabetes routine, including blood glucose testing, dietary needs, complications, and medications. This nurse can act as an advocate to help ensure the care goes smoothly.

Tips

If you have diabetes, never assume that your blood sugar will be checked regularly in the hospital. Maintain your regular blood sugar testing and do extra checks if you feel that your blood sugar may be going too high or too low.

If you have a planned surgery or treatment that will be done in the hospital and you have diabetes, read about the treatment and new medications before your hospital admission. Discuss any concerns you have with your doctor.

Some medications, such as beta-blockers for heart disease or blood pressure control, may mask symptoms of low blood sugar. When in the hospital, do not go for prolonged periods without checking your blood sugar.

Tell your nurses what symptoms you experience when you develop low blood sugar.

If your meter detects that you have low blood sugar, report this to your nurse immediately.

Fluid Problems

For people with fluid-regulation problems such as heart failure and kidney disorders, it is very important to be alert about receiving too much fluid while in the hospital. People with these conditions are generally well regulated while hospitalized; however, fluid volumes, including IVs and medications, are often tracked via manual paper systems, and the process is vulnerable to calculation errors or lost information. You may need to give frequent reminders to the doctors and nurses caring for you about this problem.

Tips

Be very alert to the amount of fluid you are receiving and the amount of fluid that you are eliminating in your urine.

At the first sign of swelling, shortness of breath, or breathing difficulty, speak to your nurse and doctor immediately.

Lung Disease

Patients with allergies, asthma, chronic obstructive pulmonary disease, emphysema, bronchitis, or other diseases related to breathing need to be very aware of new treatments, medications, and surgery. It is vital for these patients to give a thorough and complete history to their doctors and nurses when admitted to the hospital. Patients with these conditions must immediately report any breathing changes, even if they appear minor. Fluid overload and medications may affect these illnesses, and extra precautions must be taken.

Tips

If you have a respiratory illness, ask if your hospital has a special nurse case manager or other specialized nurse. If so, ask to meet with him or her so that you can review your treatments and medications.

If you are undergoing surgery, be sure to review all your lung problems with your anesthesiologist.

If you smoke and are undergoing surgery, be very accurate with your anesthesiologist about how much you smoke and for how long you have smoked. People who smoke can develop special breathing problems when undergoing anesthesia.

Neurological or Muscular Disorders

It is essential that a patient with any neurological or muscular disorder inform each of the physicians and staff members of any physical limitation. If a patient has frailty when walking, muscle weakness, a visual or hearing impairment, partial paralysis, or limitations or problems at night or other times, each new staff member should be told and reminded of these factors. It is a good idea to ask that a case manager or physical therapist be assigned to the patient to assess needs such as for physical aids or walking assistance and to evaluate the risks in the environment. This assessment can be prearranged once an admission is scheduled, or it can be arranged shortly after the patient is admitted. The patient's nurse can assist with the arrangements.

Tips

If you have a wheelchair or walker, place a tag on the item with your name and contact information. Ask the admissions clerk to log all your items onto a personal-belongings sheet. Hospitals utilize a form for this information.

If you have a chronic illness or special condition, be very alert and continually keep all the members of your health care team informed about your normal healthy routine. Do not assume that your special needs will be automatically addressed without your speaking up.

If you have had a mastectomy, remind each person taking your blood pressure, starting an IV, drawing blood, or performing any treatment to use your unaffected arm. Ask your nurse to place a sign by your bed that is visible to all health care professionals.

MASON

Joe and Rachel Williams were the proud parents of twin baby boys, Mason and Peyton. However, these Indiana parents had been through a rough course with their first child, Tyler, who had been born eight years earlier with no ability to fight infections. He had succumbed to severe combined immunodeficiency disease (SCID), also known as bubble boy syndrome, a genetic disease that manifests with a deficient immune response and the inability to fight the simplest of germs. Though Peyton was healthy, Mason also had the syndrome.

The advancements in medicine gave Joe and Rachel more hope for Mason than Tyler had been given. Dr. Joanne Kutzberg, a specialist in stem cell transplant at Duke University, explained that Mason's only chance for survival would be to undergo a special stem cell transplant. Because Mason did not have the ability to produce normal white blood cells that fight infection, the stem cell transplant was a chance for him to build a new immune system. The cells would come from the umbilical cord of a newborn baby; these cells are rich in immune response properties.

In the meantime, Mason and Peyton stayed isolated in their home. Mason was strictly protected from any outside exposure. Although Mason did not live in a bubble, neither boy was allowed to leave the home except for needed trips to the hospital. Peyton had to stay isolated so he would not carry germs to his brother. At least they had each other to play with. But even their grandparents had to wear special masks and use strict aseptic technique when visiting the boys.

A national donor search was performed and a blood cell match was found for Mason. Joe and Rachel packed up their household and took their twins to live near Duke University in North Carolina, the beginning of a long and arduous journey.

Mason had to undergo extensive chemotherapy to deplete his remaining white blood cells, which if left untouched would destroy any new transplanted stem cells. This made Mason feel sick and left him vulnerable to many kinds of illness. In addition to all the tests and tubes, he had to take other strong medications. It was a lot to endure.

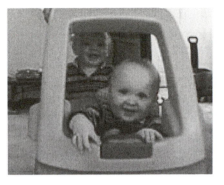

Mason and Peyton Williams. Courtesy ABC News.

In March 2002, after successful chemotherapy, the stem cells were carefully processed and administered to Mason. It would be more than a year, however, before Joe and Rachel would find out if the transplant worked. While they waited the long year, Mason had to stay in isolation with his family. He could not even go to a playground or grocery store.

With much anticipation and uncertainty, in March 2003 the Williamses met with Dr. Kutzberg to hear the final results of all of Mason's tests. His transplant had taken. Now he was able to fight off infections. The doctor told the Williamses that they should now treat little Mason like a normal child. For them, this was truly a miracle of medicine.[11]

The Future

U.S. hospitals have countless stories of miraculous healing and recovery. On one hand, the U.S. health system provides the greatest technology, most advanced medicines, and best research in the world. Health care has progressed tremendously over the last century, and the science of medicine continues to grow at an exponential rate. Yet health care is in conflict.

A commercial airline that crashed and caused 120 to 268 fatalities each day would paralyze the airline industry. The horrific incidents of jets being flown into buildings and a field brought the airline industry to its knees. If deadly airline accidents occurred every day, no one would fly; flying would be considered a foolish gamble with life. The health care industry can no longer gamble with people's lives.

Because the deaths and harm are diluted across and deep within the silence of hospitals, the problem of patient harm is not spreading across newspaper headlines every day. This dilution results in a slow progression of change.

Health leaders and consumers should do an about-face and say enough is enough. How many incidents like Jesica's and Gianni's will be tolerated? Mrs. Santillán longs for her daughter and feels the pain of that loss every day. Mr. Vargas lets dreams of playing baseball with his son slip away.

There is an urgent need to pause and take inventory. Clinicians and consumers need to come together as partners for change. It is time to listen to the patients again. They have the right to stand up and speak up for their rights and protection. They have the right to be heard. And most importantly, they have the right to be safe. The clinicians must again be willing to listen. The patient is the one who will live with the outcome of an error. The days of blind trust must end. Until the perils of error are significantly diminished, consumers need a guild to help them maneuver through the obstacles and barriers of the multilayered and unsafe systems.

The public must help to focus on the broken systems. Consumers must demand improvements in safety and lobby for legislative change. They should not cease until feasible solutions are in place. The public must know, through their partnership and use of valid data, what progress hospitals are making to design safer systems.

Physicians, nurses, pharmacists, clinicians, management, employees, and the public need to make the health care community safe for all the Bens, Alexises, Miguels, Taylors, Joses, Giannis and Jesicas of the world.

One Last Tip

Last, but not least, if you take this guide with you to the hospital and you are reading the tips, DO NOT feel intimidated by the fact that you are becoming educated and that you will speak up if you have a concern. What you say and do may save your life.

In 1998, some 600 million people traveled on commercial airliners in the United States without a single fatality. Let's endeavor for the same results in health care.

Provide knowledge to patients on the problem of error, give them tools to be safe, and partner with them in order to alter the future of health care.

APPENDIX 1

Be Safe: Preventing Medical Errors

Beware

Errors do happen. You are the best link in preventing medical and medication errors. Be Alert: Pause • Ask • Question • Confirm

Education

Before you need health care or hospital services seek information and tips about health care. Learn the basics of error prevention in case of an emergency. Learn about your illness or injury. Use health care community services or professional organizations to become educated about your condition. Talk to your doctor or health care professional about your treatments and tests.

Speak Up

Tell your doctor, your nurse, or any person giving you medicine about your ALLERGIES. Tell your doctor and health care workers about your medical history, illnesses, surgeries, and injuries. Make a written list of ALL your medicines, vitamins, herbs, and supplements. List the amounts of medicines you take and the times that you take them. Bring the list with you when you receive health care or hospital services. Keep the list current.

Act

Take action. If something is out of place, take steps to stop or fix the situation. If the situation is not resolved, ask other professionals. If something seems unusual about your medication, take action. Ask your nurse, doctor, or pharmacist.

Facts

When undergoing surgery or a procedure or going into the hospital, get the facts about what to expect. Talk to your doctor about the details of what will happen and what side effects or complications you should watch out for. Know who and when to call if something is wrong.

Error-Free

Work with patient safety groups to help reduce medical errors. Help identify hidden dangers. Tell your doctor or health care professional if you see something that causes concern. You can help to prevent medical errors.

RESOURCES

Patient Safety Resources

Anesthesia Patient Safety Foundation
4246 Colonial Park Drive
Pittsburgh, PA 15227-2621
(412) 882-8040
http://www.apsf.org/links/links.html

Bridge Medical, the Patient Safety Company
120 South Sierra Avenue
Solana Beach, CA 92075
(858) 350-0100
http://www.bridgemedical.com/index.html

To order the video "Beyond Blame," log on to
http://www.bridgemedical.com/beyond_blame.html

Centers for Disease Control
1600 Clifton Road
Atlanta, GA 30333
(800) 311-3435
http://www.cdc.gov/

Institute of Medicine
The National Academies
500 Fifth Street, NW
Washington, DC 20001
(202) 334-2138
http://www.iom.edu

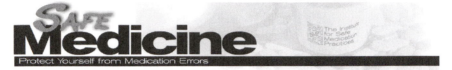

Institute for Safe Medication Practices
Huntingdon Valley, PA 19006
(215) 947-7797
http://www.ismp.org

National Patient Safety Foundation
515 N. State Street
Chicago, IL 60610
(312) 464-4848
http://npsf.org
http://www.npsf.org/html/patients.html#what

Institute of Healthcare Improvement
375 Longwood Avenue, 4th Floor
Boston, MA 02215
(617) 754-4800
http://www.ihi.org

The Leapfrog Group
c/o Academy Health
1801 K Street, NW Suite 701-L
Washington, DC 20006
(202) 292-6713
http://www.leapfroggroup.org

Joint Commission on Accreditation of Healthcare Organizations
One Renaissance Boulevard
Oakbrook Terrace, IL 60181

(630) 792-5000

http://www.jcaho.org/ptsafety_frm.html

http://www.jcaho.org

Premier Partners for a Healthier Community, Patient Safety

(877) 777-1552

http://www.premierinc.com

Sharp Healthcare

8695 Spectrum Center Blvd

San Diego, CA 92123

http://www.sharp.com/healthaz/healthinfo.cfm

VA National Center for Patient Safety

24 Frank Lloyd Wright Drive, Lobby M

PO Box 486

Ann Arbor, MI 48106-0486

(734) 930-5890

http://www.patientsafety.gov

DoctorQuality

1100 East Hector Street

Suite 6100

Conshohocken, PA 19428

(610) 828-9955

http://www.doctorquality.com/www/flash.htm

Children's Safety Resources

American Academy of Pediatrics

141 Northwest Point Boulevard

Elk Grove Village, IL 60007-1098

(847) 434-4000

http://www.aap.org/family

American Academy of Family Physicians

11400 Tomahawk Creek Parkway

Leawood, KS 66211-2672

Toll-free: (800) 274-2237

Local: (913) 906-6000

http://www.aafp.org/

The National Association of Children's Hospitals and Related Institutions (NACHRI) (provides a guide for finding children's hospitals nationwide)

http://www.childrenshospitals.net/nachri/about?/profiles_index.html

Lucile Packard Children's Hospital

Stanford University Medical Center

725 Welch Road

Palo Alto, CA 94304

(650) 497-8000

http://www.lpch.org/ForPatientsVisitors/PatientServices

Hospital and Health-Related Information

HospitalWeb—USA

http://adams.mgh.harvard.edu/hospitalwebusa.html

American Red Cross

http://www.redcross.org/faq/blooddonproc.html

American Academy of Orthopedic Surgeons

http://www.aaos.org/wordhtml/home2.htm

American Psychiatric Association

www.psych.org

WebMD

http://www.webmd.com/

Cancer Care

American Cancer Society

www.cancer.org

American Society of Clinical Oncology

www.asco.org

Diabetes

American Diabetes Association
www.diabetes.org

Heart Disease/Stroke/Vascular Disease

American Heart Association
www.americanheart.org

Physician-Related Information

American Medical Association
515 N. State Street
Chicago, IL 60610
(312) 464-5000
http://www.ama.asssn.org/

American Board of Medical Specialties (ABMS)
1007 Church Street, Suite 404
Evanston, IL 60201-5913
(866) ASK-ABMS
http://www.abms.org/member.asp

National Practitioners Data Bank
U.S. Department of Health and Human Services
U.S. Public Health Service Health Resources and Services
Administration
Division of Practitioner Data Banks
7519 Standish Place, Suite 300
Rockville, MD 20857
(301) 443-2300
http://bhpr.hrsa.gov/dqa/contactpg.htm

Federation of State Medical Boards (FSMB)
PO Box 619850
Dallas, TX 75261-9850
(817) 868-4000
http://www.fsmb.org/

Physician and Hospital Ratings

HealthGrades
http://www.healthgrades.com/

HealthScope
http://www.healthscope.org/

KEY TO PILL COMBINATIONS

The combination of pills on any one picture could seriously harm or kill a young child. Here is a guide to the photos on the last page of the color insert.

I. Top row, left to right:

1. Candy
2. Laxative
3. Candy
4. Candy
5. Acetaminophen
6. Candy

Middle row:

1. Thyroid medicine
2. Candy
3. Blood pressure medicine
4. Candy
5. Candy
6. Antidepressive medicine

Bottom row:

1. Laxative
2. Acetaminophen
3. Baby aspirin
4. Antinausea medicine
5. Narcotic
6. Candy

II. All medications (left to right):

1. Laxative
2. Laxative
3. Acetaminophen
4. Narcotic
5. Acetaminophen
6. Baby aspirin

III. From top to bottom:

1. Narcotic
2. Calcium
3. Acetaminophen
4. Candy
5. Thyroid medicine
6. Candy
7. Muscle relaxant
8. Candy

NOTES

Introduction

1. Institute of Medicine. (1999). To err is human: Building a safer health system. In Linda T. Kohn, Janet M. Corrigan, & Molla S. Donaldson (Eds.), *Errors in health care: A leading cause of death and injury* (pp. 160–184). Washington, DC: National Academy Press.

Chapter 1: The Error Factor

1. The Associated Press. (2003, 11 May). Results of teen-ager's autopsy released: Duke establishes fund to provide assistance for Hispanic patients. Retrieved 22 May 2003 from www.Journalnews.com.

2. WRAL. (2003, 21 February). Text of Duke's letter to UNOS explaining transplant mistakes. Printed with permission from Duke University Hospital, Communications and News, 19 May 2003.

3. Institute of Medicine. (1999). To err is human: Building a safer health system. In Linda T. Kohn, Janet M. Corrigan, & Molla S. Donaldson (Eds.), *Errors in health care: A leading cause of death and injury* (pp. 26–33). Washington, DC: National Academy Press.

4. Ibid.

5. Ibid.

6. Ibid.

7. Puget Sound Blood Center. Transfusion reaction, acute hemolytic. Retrieved 11 April 2003 from http://www.psbc.org/medical/transfusion.

8. Belkin, Lisa. (1997, 27 July). Health care industry, heal thyself. *The Orlando Sentinel.*

9. Institute of Medicine. (1999).

10. Zahn, Chunliu, & Miller, Marlene R. (2003, 8 October). Excess length of stay, charges and mortality attributable to medical injuries during hospitalization. *Journal of the American Medical Association, 290,* 1868–1874.

11. Institute of Medicine. (1999).

12. Reason, James. (2000, 12 March). Human error models and management. *British Medical Journal, 320,* 768–770.

13. Institute of Medicine. (1999).

14. Reason, James. (1991). *Human error.* Cambridge University Press.

15. Ibid.

16. CBSNews.com. (2003, 21 January). Health. Mastectomy mistake fuels debate. Retrieved 7 December 2003 from www.CBSNews.com.

17. Women's issues. Health hazards. (2003, 3 June). *Bodies Politic.* Retrieved 7 December 2003 from http://babelogue.citypages.com:8080/lkokmen/2003/06/03.

18. Institute of Medicine. (1999).

19. Lesar, T. S. (2001, August). Prescribing errors involving medication forms. *Journal of General Internal Medicine, 17*(8), 656–657.

20. Lazarou, J., Pomeranz, B. H., & Corey, P. N. (1998). Incidence of adverse drug reactions in hospitalized patients: A meta-analysis of prospective studies. *Journal of the American Medical Association, 279,* 1200–1205.

21. Bates, D. W., Leape, L. L., & Petrycki, S. (1993). Incidence and preventability of adverse drug events in hospitalized adults. *Journal of General Internal Medicine, 8,* 289–294.

22. Diekema, D. J., et al. (2001). Survey of infections due to staphylococcus species: Frequency of occurrence and antimicrobial susceptibility of isolates collected in the United States, Europe, and the western Pacific region for SENTRY antimicrobial surveillance program, 1997–1999. *Clinical Infectious Disease, 32* (Suppl. 2), 114–132.

23. Martone, W. J., et al. (1992). *Incidence and nature of endemic and epidemic nosocomial infections.* In J. V. Bennett & P. S. Brachman (Eds.), *Hospital infections* (pp. 577–596). Boston: Little, Brown and Company. Abstract obtained 29 March 2003 from the Centers for Disease Control, Atlanta.

24. Martone, W. J., et al. (1992). Incidence and nature of endemic and epidemic nosocomial infections. In J. V. Bennett & P. S. Brachman

(Eds.), *Hospital infections* (pp. 577–596). Abstract obtained 29 March, 2003, from the Centers for Disease Control, Atlanta.

25. Haley, R. W. (1986). Managing hospital infection control for cost-effectiveness. Chicago: American Hospital Association. Abstract obtained 29 March 2003 from the Centers for Disease Control, http://www.cdc.gov/ncidod/eid/vol7no1/kaye.htm.

26. Tye, Larry. (1999, 3 March). Patients at risk: Hospital errors. Seeking a prescription against mistakes. *The Boston Globe.*

27. Joint Commission on Accreditation of Healthcare Organizations. (2003, 7 May). Sentinel event statistics: Root causes of restraint deaths. Retrieved 3 June 2003 from http://www.JCAHO.org.

28. Ibid.

29. Institute of Medicine. (1999).

30. Midwest Business Group on Health. (2003, April). *Reducing the costs of poor-quality health care* (pp. 7–15).

31. Lazarou, Pomeranz, and Corey. (1998).

Chapter 2: Communication Vulnerabilities

1. Quality Interagency Coordination. (2000, 11 September). National summit on medical errors and patient safety research. Panel 1: Consumers and Purchasers: Testimony by Susan E. Sheridan.

2. Chassim, M. R., & Becher, E. C. (2002, 4 June). The wrong patient. *Annals of Internal Medicine, 136* (11), 826–833.

Chapter 3: Why the Silence?

1. Warsh, D. (1995). Epilogue. Lehrer, Steven. (1996). Explorers of body. *Publisher's Weekly.*

2. Ibid.

3. Institute for Safe Medication Practices. (2001). Medication safety alert. Important error prevention advisory—cisplatin over-dose, November 19, 1997. Retrieved 7 May 2002 from ismp.org.

4. Jonathan, B. (2002, 1 August). Boy lost hearing in Hopkins overdose. *The Baltimore Sun.* Retrieved 17 May 2003 from http://groups.yahoo.com/group/USA-L.

5. Dominguez, Alex. (2003, 19 December). Medical error kills young cancer patient. Retrieved 25 December 2003 from http://www.newsday.com/news/nationworld/wire/sns-ap-hopkins-potassium-death,0,4695032.story.

6. Phillips, J., et al. (2001, 1 October). Retrospective analysis of mortalities associated with medication errors. *American Journal of Health-System Pharmacy, 58,* 1835–1841.

7. Dry, L. R. (2003). Death in the radiology department. *Medico-Legal Advisor*. Retrieved 15 May 2003 from http://www.drdry.com.

8. *The Health Care Quality Improvement Act*. Public law: 99–660. (1986) 42 USC Sec. 11101 26 January 1998. Title 42: The public health and welfare. Chapter 117. *Encouraging good faith professional review*. Sec. 11101.

9. Dry, L. R. (2003).

10. Deming, W. Edwards. (1986). *Out of Crisis*. Washington, D.C.: The Edwards Deming Institute.

11. DIVISION 9. Evidence Affected or Excluded by Extrinsic Policies Chapter 1. Evidence of Character, Habit, or Custom. California Evidence Code 1157.

Chapter 4: Organized Structures within Hospitals

1. American Medical Association. Organized medical staffs. Retrieved 7 December 2003 from http://www.ama-assn.org/ama/pub/category/21.html.

2. American Medical Association. (2002). Contracts, what you should know. In *Managed care issues/Private sector advocacy*, 3rd ed. Retrieved 23 May 2003 from http://www.ama-assn.org/ama1/pub/upload/mm/368/mmcc-02-public.pdf.

Chapter 5: Who Is Watching the Hospitals?

1. Joint Commission on Accreditation of Healthcare Organizations. (2003).*Who is the joint commission on accreditation of healthcare organizations: Our mission*. Retrieved 30 March 2003 from http://www.jcaho.org/general+public/who+jc/index.htm.

2. Joint Commission on Accreditation of Healthcare Organizations. (2002, 2 April). *Joint commission to shift to unannounced surveys in 2006*. Retrieved 22 April 2003 from http://www.jcaho.org/accredited+organizations/svnp/qa_unannounced.htm.

3. Ibid.

4. Joint Commission on Accreditation of Healthcare Organizations. (2003). Frequently asked questions. Retrieved 15 April 2003 from http://www.jcaho.org/accredited+organizations/long+term+care/faqs/index.htm.

5. Joint Commission on Accreditation of Healthcare Organizations. (2002, July). *Sentinel event policy and procedures*. Retrieved 15 April 2003 from http://www.jcaho.org/accredited+organizations/hospitals/sentinel+events/reporting+alternatives.htm.

6. Institute for Safe Medication Practices. (1996, 20 November). *KCL deaths: Art imitates life.* Retrieved 18 April 2003 from http://www.ismp.org/msaarticles/art.html.

7. Ibid.

8. Stolberg, S. G. (1999, 5 December). Do no harm: Breaking down medicine's culture of silence. *New York Times.*

9. Joint Commission on Accreditation of Healthcare Organizations. (2003). Frequently asked questions.

Chapter 6: Making Safer Health Care Choices: What the Numbers Mean

1. Thomas, J. R., et al. (1996). American College of Cardiology/ American Heart Association guidelines for the management of patients with acute myocardial infarction: Executive summary. *Circulation, 94,* 2341–2350.

2. The Leapfrog Group. (2003). The Leapfrog Group fact sheet: Leapfrog's mission. Retrieved 17 May 2003 from http://leapfrog. medstat.com.

3. Young, M. O., & Birkmeyer, J. D. (2000, November/December). Potential reduction in mortality rates using an intensivist model to manage intensive care units. *Effective Clinical Practice.* Retrieved 15 April 2003 from http://www.acponline.org/journals/ecp/novdec00/ young.htm.

4. Institute for Safe Medication Practices. (2002, 18 September). Bad "marks" for order communication. ISMP handwriting. Retrieved 24 April 2003 from http://www.ismp.org/msaarticles/art.html.

5. The Leapfrog Group. (2003).

6. Young & Birkmeyer. (2000).

7. Institute of Medicine. (1999). To err is human: Building a safer health system. In Kohn, Linda T., Corrigan, Janet M., & Donaldson, Molla S. (Eds.), *Characteristics of state adverse reporting systems* (pp. 254–265). Washington, D.C.: National Academy Press.

8. Ibid.

9. Ibid.

10. Gebhart, F. (2003, 3 February). More states require reporting of drug errors. Drugtopics.com, Retrieved 19 May 2003 from drug-topics.com.

11. Millennium Health Care: Professional Development Center. (2003). *System approach to patient safety.* Retrieved 22 May 2003 from http://www.muhealth.org/~outcomes/millennium/MedErrorPBL. doc.

12. United States Pharmacopoeia. (2003). About USP. Retrieved 15 April 2003 from http://www.usp.org/aboutUSP/mission.html.

13. United States Pharmacopoeia. (2003). MEDMARX is your "must-have" solution to medication error prevention. Retrieved 25 April 2002 from http://www.usp.org.

14. Institute for Safe Medication Practices. (2003). About the Institute for Safe Medication Practices. Retrieved 3 May 2003 from http://www.ismp. org/Pages/about.html.

15. United States Pharmacopoeia. (2003). Medication error reporting program: Summary. Retrieved 25 April 2003 from http://www.usp.org.

Chapter 7: Rapid Advancements in Medicine

1. The inventive spirit. http://www.philalandmarks.org/page_houses/physick/history/phys_history.html.

2. Chassim, M. (1998). Is health care ready for six-sigma quality? *Milbank Quarterly, 76*, 510, 565–591.

3. Lester, K. (2003, March). The growth in dispensing errors and its effect. Retrieved 13 May 2003 from http://www.kirbylester.com.

4. Institute for Safe Medication Practices. (2003, 17 April). "Looks" like a problem. Ephedrine and epinephrine. Retrieved 20 April 2003 from http://www.ismp.org/msaarticles/looksprint.htm.

5. Gravenstein, J. S. (1995, Fall). How safe is "safe"? *Anesthesia Patient Safety Foundation Newsletter.* Retrieved 14 April 2003 from http://www.ahcpr.gov/news/ulp/errors/ulpmeder4.htm.

6. Siker, E. S. (2003). Special article: A safety tutorial? Anesthesia Patient Safety Foundation. Retrieved 8 May 2003 from http://www. gas net.org/societies/apsf/newsletter/1989/summer/index.html#art%203.

7. Anesthesia Patient Safety Foundation. (2003). Mission. Retrieved 22 May 2003 from http://www.gasnet.org/societies/apsf/mission.php.

8. Pierce, Ellison C. Enhancing patient safety from 1980s through the present. Anesthesia Patient Safety Foundation.

9. Siker. (2003).

10. Ornstein, C. (2003, 24 February). Infant anesthesia problems spark debate. *Kaiser Papers.* Retrieved 22 May 2003 from http://www.kaiserpapers.org/debate.html.

Chapter 8: Old Designs, Prone to Errors: System Failures and Human Factors

1. Reason, James. (1990). *Human error.* Cambridge, MA: Cambridge University Press.

2. Newsday.com. (2002, 8 February). Tragic error. Retrieved 30 March 2003 from http://www.newsday.com/search/dispatcher.front?Query=gianni+vargas&target=article.

3. Smetzer, Judy L. (1998, May). Lesson from Colorado: Beyond blaming individuals. *Nursing, 98.*

4. Adams, Damon. (2001, 28 May). Robert Wood Johnson Foundation programs aim at cutting medical errors. *AMNews.* Retrieved 19 May 2003 from http://www.ama-assn.org/amednews/2001/05/28/prsd0528.htm - 16.2KB.

5. Singer, Sara, & Gaba, David. (2003, 8 April). *Discrepancies in perceptions of patient safety.* Center for Health Policy, Center for Primary Care and Outcome Research. http://chppcor.stanford.edu/news/pr/4-8-03-PS.html.

6. Shepherd, William. (2001, 23 October). Human factors issues in aircraft maintenance. *Federal Air Surgeon's Medical Bulletin.* http://www2.faa.gov/avr/aam/fasb597/23.htm.

7. Lindsey T. (2001, June 28). *Beyond blame.* Solano Beach, CA: Bridge Medical.

8. American Medical Association. (2003). What are the residents' work conditions? Retrieved 14 May 2003 from http://www.ama-assn.org/ama/pub/category/7570.html.

9. Leape, L. L. (1994). Error in medicine. *Journal of the American Medical Association, 272* (23),1851–1857.

10. Manrique, Alverto; Valdivia, Juan Carlos; & Jimenez, Alfonso. (2003). Human factor engineering applied to nuclear power plant design. San Sebastian de los Reyes, Madrid 28709 Spain. (TECNATOM, S.A.). Retrieved 28 April 2003 from http://www3.inspi.ufl.edu/icapp03/program/abstracts/3337.html.

11. Stone, Fred. (2001). Medical team management: Using teamwork to prevent medical errors. (Legal Medicine). Retrieved 15 April 2003 from http://www.ufip.org/Departments/legalmed/legmed2001/medical.htm.

12. Institute of Medicine. (1999). To err is human: Building a safer health system. In Linda T. Kohn, Janet M. Corrigan, & Molla S. Donaldson (Eds.), *Errors in health care: A leading cause of death and injury* (pp. 26–33). Washington, DC: National Academy Press.

13. Gaba, David. (2003). Simulation center. VA Palo Alto Health Care System. http://anesthesia.stanford.edu/VASimulator/simcntr.htm.

14. Weinger, Matthew. (2003). Center for Healthcare Simulation. San Diego, CA. http://simcenter.ucsd.edu/.

15. Berens, Michael J. (2000, 6 December). Watchdog gets tough on hospital IV devices. *Chicago Tribune.*

16. Carstensen, Peter B. (2003). Program plan: Implications for the medical device industry. Division of User Programs and Systems Analysis, Office of Health and Industry Programs, Center for Devices and Radiological Health, Food and Drug Administration. Retrieved 8 April 2003 from http://www.fda.gov/cdrh/humanfactors/whatis.html.

17. Ibid.

Chapter 9: Disclosure

1. Leapfrog Group. (2003). *The Leapfrog Group fact sheet: Leapfrog's mission.* Retrieved 17 May 2003 from http://leapfrog. medstat.com.

2. Loecher, B., & Boyer, P. (2001, 21 January). Get out of the hospital alive. *Prevention, 105–109, 159–161.*

3. Dateline NBC. MSNBC News. (2001, 1 January). A deadly mistake. Retrieved 1 April 2003 from http://stacks.msnbc.com/news/657566.asp?cp1=1.

4. Bridge Medical. *Beyond Blame.* Solano Beach, CA.

5. Kraman, S. S., & Hamm, G. (1999, 21 December). Risk management: Extreme honesty may be the best policy. *Annals of Internal Medicine, 131,* 963–967.

6. Ibid.

7. Loecher & Boyer. (2001).

8. Kraman & Hamm. (1999).

9. Wilborn, T. (2001, March/April). VA patient safety program shows promise. *Disabled American Veterans Magazine.* http://www.dav.org/magazine/2001–2/VA_Patient_Safet1680.html.

10. Ibid.

11. Adams, D. (2001, 23 July). Held accountable: New rules require hospitals to tell patients about mistakes. *AMNews.* Retrieved 22 April 2003 from http://www.ama-assn.org/sci-pubs/amnews/pick_01/prsb0723.htm.

12. Institute for Safe Medication Practices. (2001, 22 August). ISMP survey on perceptions of a non-punitive culture produces some surprising results. Retrieved 22 April 2003 from http://www.ismp.org/MSAarticles/nonpunitive.html.

13. United States Court of Appeals for the Federal Circuit. (1996, 23 October). 95–3732, Dennis Dunn & Frank Ruiz vs. Department of Veterans Affairs. http://www.law.emory.edu/fedcircuit/oct96/95-3732.html.

14. Office of Personnel Management. The federal government's human resource agency. EAP programs. http://www.opm.gov/ehs/eappage.asp.

15. Landro, Linda. (2003, 25 March). Hospitals encourage staff to report medical errors. *The Wall Street Journal.*

16. Hadley, Jeffery. (2003). *An online reporting system for traffic safety.* Unpublished manuscript. National Study Center for Trauma and Emergency Medical Systems. University of Maryland, School of Medicine. http://www.accident-report.org/faq.html.

17. Harvard University's John F. Kennedy School of Government and the Council for Excellence in Government. "Close call." Dr. James Bagaian. Retrieved 19 May 2003 from http://www.ksg.harvard.edu/.

18. The Coalition to Heal Healthcare in Florida. (2003). *Reporting near misses.* Retrieved 20 May 2003 from http://heal-fl-health-care-pdf.netcomsus.com/presskit_2003legislativeplan.pdf.

Chapter 10: Beyond Medical Malpractice

1. Albert, Tanya. (2003, 13 May). Illinois physicians demand immediate tort reform at rally. *American Medical News.* Retrieved 19 May 2003 from http://www.ama-assn.org/ama/pub/article/9255-7662.html.

2. Ramachandran, Raghu. (2003, 21 January). Did investments affect medical malpractice premiums? *Insurance Asset Management.* Brown Bros. Harriman. Retrieved 28 June 2004 from http://salsa.bbh.com/news/archives/000283.php?insurance=1.

3. Wilbourn, S. L. Testimony before joint hearing of Congress on medical litigation. February 11, 2003.

4. American Medical Association. (2003, 3 March). *New AMA analysis shows 18 states now in full-blown medical liability crisis.*

5. Albert, Tanya. (2003, 3 March). Doctors rally against rising liability rates. *AMNews.* http://www.ama-assn.org/amednews/2003/03/03/prsa0303.htm.

6. The Foundation for Taxpayers and Consumer Rights. (2003). Insurance industry reform, not liability limits, lowered and stabilized insurance rates in California. Retrieved 20 May 2003 from http://www.consumerwatchdog.org/healthcare/medmal.php.

7. Americans for Insurance Reform. (2003, January). Medical malpractice stable/loss unstable rates in West Virginia. Retrieved 18 May 2003 from http://www.insurance-reform.org/StableLossesWV.pdf.

8. Public Citizen. (2002, 30 July). Letter from Public Citizen in opposition to the McConnell Medical Malpractice Amendment. Retrieved 28 June 2004 from http://www.citizen.org/congress/civjus/medmal/articles.cfm?ID=8100.

9. McDougal, Linda. (2003, 11 February). Testimony before Patient Access Crisis: The Role of Medical Litigation Bill Number H.R.

5: Joint Hearing. Retrieved 2 April 2003 from http://health.senate.gov/testimony/009 _tes.html.

10. Becker, Paul, president of the Citizens for a Sound Economy. http://thomas.loc.gov/cgi-bin/query/F?c108:1:./temp/~c108 VYQ3jb:e2156.

11. HR. 5 Health Efficient, Accessible, Low Cost, Timely Health Act of 2003 (HEALTH). 108th Congress, 2nd Session. Retrieved 20 August 2004 from http://www.aafp.org/x19669.xml?printxml.

12. The Journal News, New York (28 March 2003). Limiting malpractice awards needs exception. The Foundation for Taxpayers and Consumer Rights. http://www.consumerwatchdog.org/healthcare/nw/nw003224.php3.

13. Glass, B. (2000, August). Case results and verdicts: Fredericksburg jury awards $305,000 in medication error case. Retrieved 19 May 2003 from http://www.vamedmal.com/case_results.cfm#31.

14. History of the Long Term Care Ombudsman programs. (1998). Georgia LTCO training manual 1998. Retrieved 12 May 2003 from http://teampublish.allsoldout.net/teampubv3/includes/aLTCOProgramtext.pdf.

15. E-Health Care Mediations. Inc. (2003). Collaborative solutions for clinical conflict. Retrieved 29 April 2003 from http://www.wiley.com/WileyCDA/WileyTitle/productCd-CRQ.html.

16. Ahearn, Michael. (2001, December 1). Medical malpractice arbitration. Widener University School of Law Alternative Dispute Resolution Seminar, Harrisburg, PA.

17. Shapiro, J. P. (2000, 17 July). Taking the mistakes out of medicine: Minnesota Children's remakes its culture in the name of safety. *U.S. News and World Report.*

18. Albert, T. (2002, 11 February). One physician hopes legal insurance could be one way to help halt the medical malpractice crisis. *AMNews.* Retrieved 18 April 2003 from http://www.ama-assn.org/sci-pubs/amnews/pick_02/prl20211.htm.

Chapter 11: Toward a New Safety Culture: How the Change Will Happen

1. The Hall of Public Service. (1991, 16 February). Ralph Nader Consumer Crusader Interview. Washington, D.C. Retrieved 3 May 2003 from http://www.achievement.org/autodoc/page/nad0int-1.

2. National Highway Traffic Safety Administration. (2003). About the National Highway Traffic Safety Administration.

Retrieved 15 April 2003 from http://www.nhtsa.dot.gov/nhtsa/whatis/overview.

3. Chin, Tyler. (2003, 8 September). What is an EMR? *AMNews.* Retrieved 4 December 2003 from http://www.ama-assn.org/amednews/2003/09/08/bise0908.htm.

4. Gabriel, Barbara. (2002, February). It's a wired world: Information technology enhancing patient care. Association of American Medical Colleges. Retrieved 3 May 2003 from http://www.aamc.org/newsroom/reporter/feb02/wiredworld.htm.

5. Gabriel. (2002).

6. Boodman, Sandra G. (2002, 3 December). No end to errors. *The Washington Post,* p. HE01. Retrieved 15 April 2003 from http://www.washingtonpost.com/ac2/wp-dyn/A58443-2002Nov30?language=print.

7. *Federal Register 69,* no. 38, 9119. (26 February 2004). Accessed via Federal Register Online, wais.access.gpo.gov, DOCID:fr26Fe04-24.

8. Hawryluk, Markian. (2004, 15 March). FDA targets medication errors by requiring bar coding on drugs. *AMNews.* Retrieved 27 June 2004 from http://www.ama-assn.org/amednews/2004/03/15/gvl10315.htm.

9. Zwillich, Todd. (2004). Bush pushes for electronic medical records expansion. *Government and Law.* Retrieved 27 June 2004 from http://www.drugtopics.com/be_core/content/journals/d/data/2004/0517/d3record05b.html.

Chapter 12: The Patient Partnership: What Needs to Change

1. Institute of Medicine. (2001). *Crossing the quality chasm: A new health system for the 21st century* (p. 67). Washington, D.C.: National Academy Press.

2. Midwest Business Group on Health. (2003, April). *Reducing the costs of poor-quality health care* (pp. 7–15). Chicago: Midwest Business Group on Health.

3. Kizer, Kenneth W. (2000, 9 February). Testimony before the House Committee on Commerce, Subcommittee on Health and Environment and Subcommittee on Oversight and Investigations. House Committee on Veterans Affairs, Subcommittee on Health. Hearing on Medical Errors: Improving Quality of Care and Consumer Information.

4. Institute of Medicine. (1999). To err is human: Building a safer health system. In Linda T. Kohn, Janet M. Corrigan, & Molla S. Donaldson (Eds.), *Errors in health care: A leading cause of death and injury* (pp. 26–33). Washington, DC: National Academy Press.

5. Nelson, K., Kivlahan, C., & Buddenbaum, J. (2002, September). The development of an electronic voluntary adverse event reporting system. *Business Briefing: Next Generation HealthCare: The Official Publication of the World Medical Association.*

6. Liberto, Jennifer. (2003, 19 April). Suit says doctor botched surgery. *St. Petersburg Times.* Retrieved 15 May 2003 from http://www. sptimes.com/2003/04/19/Hernando/Suit_says_doctor_botc. shtml.

7. Gallagher, Thomas H., Waterman, Amy D., Ebers, Alison G., Fraser, Victoria J., & Levinson, Wendy. (2003, February). Patients' and physicians' attitudes regarding the disclosure of medical errors. *Journal of the American Medical Association, 289,* 1001–1007.

8. Institute for Safe Medication Practices. (2002, 18 September). Bad "marks" for order communication. Retrieved 1 May 2003 from http://www. ismp.org/msaarticles/badprint.htm.

9. Keller, James. (2003, 5 May). Letter to editor. *Nurseweek, 5.*

10. McCormack, John and Catherine. (2000). Our little angel, Taylor McCormack's story. Patient stories. Retrieved 15 May 2003 from http://www.memorial2taylor.com/.

11. Agency for Healthcare Research and Quality. (2004, 7 June). Children in hospitals frequently experience medical injuries. Press release. Retrieved 27 June 2004 from http://www.ahcpr.gov/ news/press/.

12. Norton, Amy. (2003, March 4). Report details errors in hospitalized kids. *Reuter's Health.* Retrieved 15 May 2003 from http://www.reutershealth.com/en/index.html.

13. American Academy of Pediatrics. (2001, June). Policy statement. Principles of patient safety in pediatrics. (RE060027). National Initiative for Children's Health Care Quality Project Advisory Committee. 107(6). Retrieved 11 May 2003 from http://www.aap. org/policy/re060027.html.

14. Woodhull, Paula. (28 May 2004). Governor signs Taylor's Law. *Pembroke Mariner.* Retrieved 27 June 2004 from http://www. townonline.com/pembroke/news/local_regional/pem_newpetay lorslaw05262004.htm.

15. Institute of Medicine. (1999).

16. American Medical Association. (2002, 8 May). Statement to House Energy and Commerce Subcommittee on Health, "Reducing medical errors: A review of innovative strategies to improve patient safety."

17. Ibid.

18. McCormack & McCormack. (2000).

19. Ibid.

20. Ibid.

21. Centers for Disease Control. (2004). Public health bills. Patient safety. Retrieved 29 June 2004 from http://www.cdc.gov/washington/pbhlbill/patntsaf.htm.

Chapter 13: Hospitals on the Mend

1. Agency for Healthcare Research and Quality: Reauthorization fact sheet. Retrieved 15 April 2003 from http://www.ahcpr.gov/about/ahrqfact.htm.

2. Institute for Safe Medication Practices. (2000). ISMP survey medication errors. Retrieved 30 April 2003 from http://www.ismp.org/MSAarticles/nonpunitive.html.

3. Institute of Medicine Board of Health Care Services. (2003). *Patient safety: Achieving a new standard of care.* Washington, DC: National Academy Press.

4. Institute of Medicine. (2004). Keeping patients safe, transforming the work environment of nurses. In Ann Page (Ed.), *Maximizing Workforce Capability* (pp. 163–184). Washington, DC: National Academy Press.

5. Pittsburgh Regional Health Care Initiative. (1999, December). Charter agreement. Retrieved 30 April 2003 from http://www.prhi.org/pdfs/coalition/hospital_charter000613.pdf.

6. The San Diego Center for Patient Safety (SDCPS) is a collaborative effort between the Veterans Affairs (VA) San Diego Healthcare System and the University of California–San Diego, Health Sciences. Retrieved 23 April 2003 from http://health.ucsd.edu/news/2001/11_01_Weinger. html.

7. Ibid.

8. National Center for Education Statistics. (1992). The 1992 national adult literacy survey: Overview. Retrieved 3 May 2003 from http://nces.ed.gov/naal/design/about92.asp.

9. Healthy People 2010. Healthy people. Retrieved 3 May 2003 from http://www.healthypeople.gov/default.htm. *Modern Healthcare Daily Dose EXTRA.*

Chapter 14: What You Can Do to Protect Yourself

1. American Medical Association. (2003, 21 January—updated). Policy H-165.896 (7). Report 2 of the Council on Scientific Affairs (I-

98). Physician education of their patients about prescription medicines.

2. WebMD. Who we are. Retrieved 15 May 2003 from http://my.webmed. com/who_we_are/about_webmd/default.htm.

3. WebMD. Retrieved 29 June 2004 from http://my.webmd. com/content/article/71/81349.htm?lastselect edguid={5FE84E90-BC77-4056-A91C-9531713CA348.

4. Patient Rights Program. (2003). *Rights at your fingertips.* Boston: Health Law Department of the Boston University School of Public Health.

5. McKenzie, John. (2001, 8 May). Misdiagnosing cancer: Patients should always consult a second opinion. ABC News. Retrieved 13 April 2003 from http://abcnews.go.com/sections/ wnt/WorldNewsTonight/wnt010508_misdiagnosing_cancer_ feature.html.

6. National Patient Safety Foundation at the American Medical Association: Public Opinion of Patient Safety Issues. Survey conducted by Louis Harris & Associates, September 1997.

7. McGlynn, E. A., et al. (2003, 26 June). The quality of health care delivered to adults in the United States. *New England Journal of Medicine, 348*, 2635-2645.

8. Patient Rights Program. (2003).

9. American Medical Association. (1992, June). Policy E-8.041, Second Opinion. Retrieved 3 May 2003 from http://www.ama-assn.org/ama/pub/category/8475.html.

10. Shaw, Susan. (2003, 31 March). *Errors: Diabetes care.* Diabetes interview.

11. ABC News. (2004, 29 August). Medical miracle, toddler battles "bubble boy syndrome." Retrieved 18 January 2004 from *ABC News,* http://abcnews.go.com/sections/2020/Living/2020_mason williams030829.html.

SELECT BIBLIOGRAPHY

Harvard Public Health Review. (2000). *The human factor.* Retrieved 14 April 2003 from http://www.hsph.harvard.edu/review/review.

Helmreich, R. L., & Merritt, A. (1998). *Culture at work in aviation and medicine: National, organizational and professional influences.* Brookfield, VT: Ashgate.

Joint Commission on Accreditation of Healthcare Organizations. (2003, July). Sentinel event policy and procedures. Revised (electronic version). Oakbrook Terrace, IL: http://www.JCAHO.org.

McWhinny, Bruce D. (1998, January). *Reducing the human and economic costs of drug therapy complications.* Dublin, OH: Cardinal Health.

Prager, Linda O. (1999, 22–29 November). Jury blames doctor's bad penmanship for patient death. *AMNews.*

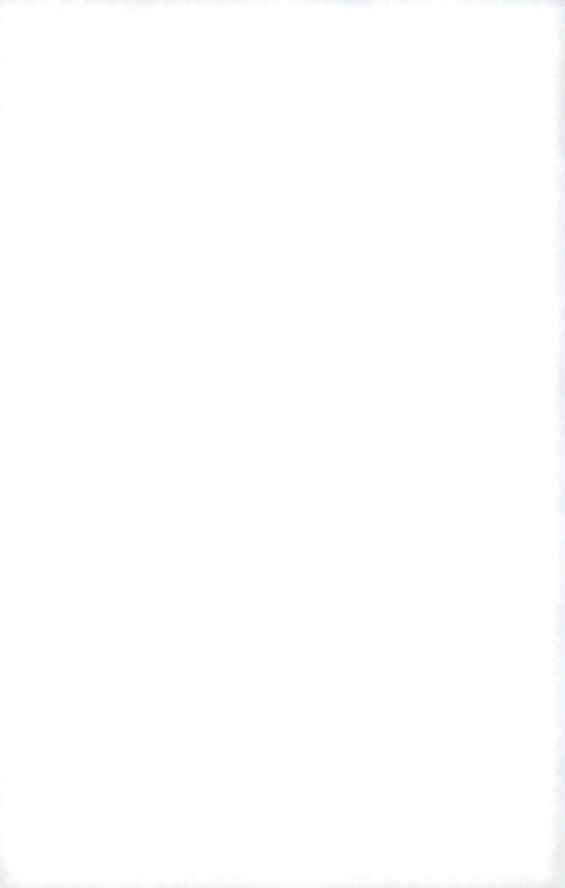

INDEX

About the Author

KARIN JANINE BERNTSEN is Vice President of Patient Safety and Quality Improvement at a large southern California health care system. She has worked in the hospital and health care system for more than 25 years. Her current role includes the implementation of patient safety, medical error review, hospital policy setting, medical staff responsibility, infection control oversight and quality improvement. As a registered nurse, she has worked in emergency, critical care, and cardiac care units.